LIVING WELL
WITH PARKINSON'S

LIVING WELL
WITH PARKINSON'S

SECOND EDITION

Glenna Atwood

with

Lila Green Hunnewell and Roxanne Moore Saucier

Foreword by Robert G. Feldman, M.D.
Professor and Chairman Emeritus, Department of Neurology
Boston University School of Medicine

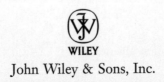

WILEY

John Wiley & Sons, Inc.

Published by John Wiley & Sons, Inc., Hoboken, New Jersey
Published simultaneously in Canada

The information contained in this book is not intended to serve as a replacement for professional medical advice. Any use of the information in this book is at the reader's discretion. The author and the publisher specifically disclaim any and all liability arising directly or indirectly from the use or the application of any information contained in this book. A health-care professional should be consulted regarding your specific situation.

For general information about our other products and services, please contact our Customer Care Department within the United States at (800) 762-2974, outside the United States at (317) 572-3993 or fax (317) 572-4002.

Wiley also publishes its books in a variety of electronic formats. Some content that appears in print may not be available in electronic books. For more information about Wiley products, visit our web site at www.wiley.com.

Library of Congress Cataloging-in-Publication Data:

Atwood, Glenna Wotton, date.
    Living well with Parkinson's / Glenna Atwood, with Lila Green
Hunnewell and Roxanne Moore Saucier / foreword by Robert G.
Feldman.—Second edition
      p. cm.
    Includes bibliographical references and index.
    ISBN 0-471-28223-5 (pbk.)
    1. Atwood, Glenna Wotton, date. 2. Parkinson's disease—Popular
works. I. Hunnewell, Lila Green. II. Saucier, Roxanne Moore, date.
III. Title.
    RC382.A88 2005
    616.8'33—dc22

                                       2004028305

Printed in the United States of America

10 9 8 7 6 5 4 3 2 1

To Blaine, my love

CONTENTS

Foreword

Glenna Atwood shared her experiences and insights about how she and her family coped with Parkinson's disease in the first edition of *Living Well with Parkinson's*.

Her words were educational and inspirational to many people affected by this intrusion in their life's plan. Glenna, with Blaine—her husband and best friend—have spoken to audiences throughout North America, sharing information on how to get the most out of their doctor, their medications, and each day of their lives. The inevitable progression of Parkinson's disease in Glenna provided more challenges to meet and deal with for the Atwoods. One problem encountered by patients is simply getting older and living with concurrent illnesses. In addition to Parkinson's, Glenna had a cardiac condition, which eventually caused her death. The second edition of this book includes her ideas and insights on living with advanced Parkinson's disease.

Each person with Parkinson's has his or her unique experiences, which require an individually tailored plan. What is universal in Parkinson's disease is the need for each person to learn and understand as much as possible about this condition, as this knowledge leads to more effective coping, proper management, and therapeutic success. This second edition of *Living Well with Parkinson's* provides invaluable information about the many additional medications, surgical interventions, and nutritional and physical therapy approaches that have been introduced for the care of patients with Parkinson's since the landmark discovery of levodopa. Armed with lessons learned from physicians, nurses, and other patients, people affected by Parkinson's need not be victims of the process.

—Robert G. Feldman, M.D.
Chairman Emeritus, Department of Neurology,
Professor of Neurology, Pharmacology,
and Public Health,
Boston University School of Medicine,
Director, American Parkinson Disease
Association Advanced Center for Research
at Boston University,
Medical Director, APDA Information and
Referral Center

Preface to the Second Edition

For those of you who already know that Glenna passed away, as well as for people who are meeting her for the first time in this book, I would like to share a little of her story.

Glenna had Parkinson's for about twenty years but never gave up living. A year after her diagnosis, she retired from teaching so that we could do some of the things we had planned for later in life.

We financed a motor home and traveled to many places in this country that we had always wanted to see. In fact, Glenna wrote most of the first edition of this book while we were on the road. She usually wrote in the morning while her medicine was most effective.

We talked about ideas, and she wrote while I drove. This was great for her, because we could plan the day around how she felt, with no phone calls or other interruptions.

As a result of the public response to the first edition, we were asked to speak to groups throughout most of the United States and parts of Canada. Again, we traveled by motor home, this time visiting people who had written to Glenna after reading the book.

She was always eager to go to the mailbox to discover who had written to her, and from where. She received letters not only from people in the United States but from those living in Europe and as far away as Australia and New Zealand. Glenna always tried to answer each letter.

As you will see, she didn't let Parkinson's get her down. In fact, we worked on the book's revision in a campground in Florida. She and I still ran the Parkinson's support group that we started more than eighteen years ago. She remained busy on committees, in church, and by planning special events with her grandchildren. They were her pride and joy.

It wasn't Parkinson's but other health problems that limited Glenna at the end. In fact, she died of a heart attack.

She was the greatest of copilots. I always told her that she made my world go around.

Be like Glenna—try to live your life to the fullest.

—Blaine Atwood

Preface to the First Edition

This is the book that I wish I could have found when my Parkinson's was diagnosed in 1981. At the time, very little information was available for the layperson, and the little that existed was very depressing. What I wanted to find was a source of information that would help me understand Parkinson's, that would give me an opportunity to relate to someone who has managed well in the same situation, and that would leave me with reasons to maintain a positive attitude.

This is my personal story: how I have coped and how I continue to cope positively as a person living with Parkinson's. It is interwoven with facts about managing Parkinson's as I have learned them since my diagnosis, through

- Evaluating my own experiences
- Reading the current scientific literature
- Attending workshops, conferences, and symposia
- Participating actively in a support group
- Talking with other people who have Parkinson's

My Parkinson's specialist, Dr. Robert G. Feldman, and his knowledgeable team in the Parkinson's Program at Boston Medical

Center (which is affiliated with Boston University School of Medicine) have also contributed significantly to my education.

In this book, I attempt to present the facts while, at the same time, sharing the ups and downs of my daily life as someone who has Parkinson's. I could not share my story without also relating some of the experiences of my family and friends, since they are so much a part of my life.

My hope is that all people with Parkinson's will find hope and guidance here: that this book may encourage them to say, "Here is a person who has had Parkinson's for twenty years, and she and her family are living happy, productive lives. If she can do it, I can do it."

Parkinson's is a progressive disease. A cure is yet to be found. But with current medications and therapies, and the proper personal care, there is reason to believe that a person with Parkinson's can live a satisfying life. New medications and other scientific breakthroughs are making a great impact on the quality of our lives while we await the cure.

Acknowledgments

I wish to express special gratitude to:

My Parkinson's specialist, Dr. Robert G. Feldman, the head of the Department of Neurology at Boston University School of Medicine, who inspired me to write this book and who graciously consented to write a foreword for it;

Lila Hunnewell, who collaborated with me in the writing of this book;

Cathi Thomas, R.N., M.S., the coordinator of the American Parkinson Disease Association (APDA) Information and Referral Center, and a member of "the Parkinson's team" at Boston Medical Center, who read the manuscript and made suggestions for its improvement;

Judith Green, Ph.D., a professor and the chair of the Psychology Department at William Paterson College of New Jersey, who kept Lila Hunnewell and me informed of the latest medical and scientific research pertaining to Parkinson's disease and who contributed several tasty recipes to the chapter on nutrition; and

Glennis Sherwood, my friend and neighbor, who took the time, despite a very busy schedule, to type the early copies of the manuscript.

* * *

The authors are grateful for the use of the following materials:

"Living with Parkinson's: What You Can Do for Yourself," by Mark Flapan, Ph.D., from the *PDF Newsletter*, reprinted with permission from the Parkinson's Disease Foundation, New York, NY, Autumn, 1989.

Excerpts from an untitled essay by George W. Paulson, M.D., and Joseph L. Howard, from UPF *Newsletter*, 1985, no. 4, part 2, quoted with permission from the United Parkinson Foundation, 360 West Superior Street, Chicago, IL 60610.

Excerpt from "Mirror, Mirror on the Wall," by Ellen Levin, quoted with permission from Parkinson's Educational Program (PEP-USA), 3900 Birch Street, Newport Beach, CA 92660. (Undated flyer.)

Excerpt from "Swallowing Problems," in *Speech Problems and Swallowing Problems in Parkinson's Disease*, quoted with the permission of the American Parkinson Disease Association, 60 Bay Street, Staten Island, NY 10301. (Undated.)

Excerpt from *Love You Forever*, © Robert Munsch, published by Firefly Books, Ltd., Willowdale, Ontario, Canada, 1986.

"Signed and Sealed," from *I Am So Glad You Married Me*, by Lois Wyse, published by American Greetings, Cleveland, Ohio, 1972. Quoted with permission from Lois Wyse.

Note

The text for chapter 8, "Medications and Therapies," is based on a search of medical and scientific literature conducted by the authors and may not reflect the views or the practice methods of Dr. Feldman or his medical team at Boston Medical Center.

CHAPTER 1

Do Not Disturb!

Things are good right now,
Really good.
So if you find a
"Do Not Disturb" sign,
Hang it outside
The door to my life.

—*Lois Wyse*, I Am So Glad You Married Me

Life was beautiful in 1978. My marriage was solid, and my husband and I felt better than ever about our relationship. We were pleased with our children, now grown and married to individuals whom we loved dearly. My career as an educator was at its peak, and I felt very productive. I was forty-seven years old. Physically, I had never felt better. I had wonderful friends and relatives. I had a lovely home in Maine. Is it any wonder that I did not want anything to disturb my life?

I was born Glenna Wotton in 1931, in a small community in northern Maine. I grew up during the Depression years, surrounded by relatives who were short on money but never short on love and caring for one another. Mine was a secure world, where life revolved around the one-room school, the church, and my family. Eventually, when I left home to become a teacher, I was armed with faith and the values with which I had grown up.

At the University of Maine in Farmington, I earned my B.S. in Home Economics, and I met Blaine Atwood, who was also preparing to teach. We married and settled in Hampden, not far from Bangor, and near Orono, where we could continue our education while we taught school. Eventually, I became a teacher and then the chairman of the Home Economics Department of Hampden Academy.

Those were active, exciting years. I expanded the home economics program to include courses in consumer education, independent living, family life, and child development, and I started a nursery school within the department. The Maine Department of Education was using some of my courses as models, and other school systems in Maine, other states, and even other nations, were adapting my course, "Independent Living." It was a good feeling to be contacted by people who wanted to use my ideas. In 1975, I was named Maine's "Home Economics Teacher of the Year."

I looked forward to a blissful future. There were so many things to enjoy and accomplish. For one thing, I assumed we would have grandchildren. I planned to be the happiest, peppiest grandmother: my grandchildren would never have to deal with a grumpy, pokey old lady. I would retire early from the school system and embark on an enterprise of my own. I considered many possibilities. I could run my own school, where there would be no bells to require my students to jump up and leave before they were ready. I could start a day-care center based on ideas I believed in. I had ideas for at least fifty pursuits, but I hadn't made a choice. I felt that, eventually, God would help me choose.

Was it on July 3, 1978, on December 24, 1979, or on some other date that I first felt a change? I really can't say. I do know that "it" sneaked up on me as I went on my way. Once in a while, my right arm felt clumsy as I walked or stood, as if I didn't know what to do with it. But I ignored it. Doesn't everyone feel a bit awkward once in a while? At times, Blaine lost patience with my pace when we were walking and asked me to speed up. He complained that if he slowed down for me, I would slow down even more. I assumed that this was Blaine's problem, not mine: he was always in a hurry.

Then one day in the summer of 1980, while I was writing a letter to my daughter, Susan, my fingers became balky. The smooth flow of my writing was lost. I was annoyed but said nothing. This feeling in my hands did not go away, and it took me longer and longer to write anything. Sometimes I had to draw the letters or print. My letter-writing habits began to change: I wrote shorter and shorter letters. But I thought, "Ignore this change! Eventually, it will go away."

School reopened, and things were almost back to normal, yet I continued to be nagged by physical problems: Why was I getting so tired? Why was I really dragging by noon? What were the weird sensations I felt from time to time? My legs especially seemed to feel strange and heavy: they jerked or felt as if a rubber band were around them. But I felt that I must not complain; if I didn't tell anyone, these sensations would go away. I remembered the time, many years ago, when I learned that my fifteen-month-old niece had been struck and killed by a car, I had *screamed*, telling myself that if I screamed loudly enough, the news would not be true. This time I hoped that silence would work. Although I had spent years teaching students to be open about their feelings, I kept all this to myself.

Early in 1981, I caught the flu. My recovery was very slow, and finally my daughter, Susan, and my husband, Blaine, insisted that I go to a doctor. Coincidentally, I had just been reading a medical column in the daily newspaper, in which a reader had asked about the symptoms of Parkinson's disease. The doctor's answer described my symptoms: "The earliest signs are apt to be a difficulty in handwriting, a slight trembling of the hand, and a jackknife effect when you put two fingers together." Overcome by anxiety, I knew, but I still didn't tell anyone about my symptoms. I still hoped I was wrong. Yet I knew the time had come to see a doctor. Without telling my family, I admitted to myself that the problem was bigger than a simple case of the flu. One thing at a time.

I made an appointment for March 30 with my family doctor. After the usual physical examination and discussion of my symptoms, my doctor said he suspected I might have Parkinson's disease. He happened to have a young student doctor in his office who was preparing to specialize in neurology. My doctor called him in, told him my symptoms, and said he suspected Parkinson's. The student observed my tremor and asked me to walk. My walk was awkward, and my arm swing was almost nonexistent. His statement was cold and brief: "That isn't Parkinson's. The tremor is too fine. I'd say it's more likely to be a tumor on the brain." With that, he left. I do not know his name, but whoever he is, and wherever he is, I hope he has learned a great deal more about diagnosing Parkinson's and about dealing with patients.

In the absence of any definitive diagnostic test for Parkinson's, my doctor called to make an appointment for me with a neurologist in Bangor. But this was March, and the neurologist couldn't give me an appointment until July. After all, what's a three- or four-month delay when you are waiting to hear whether you have Parkinson's disease or a brain tumor?

Blaine and I were thankful that my doctor did not want to wait until July. He offered to contact a neurologist in Boston, if we were willing to travel that far. We were, and an appointment in Boston was made for the following week.

During that week, we tried to go on as usual, to work, to sleep, and to eat. At the time, one of our very dear friends was dying of a cancerous tumor on the brain, and our anxiety about the possibility of a tumor on my brain was almost unbearable.

Blaine and I took Friday off and journeyed to Boston to see my first neurologist. This doctor was a mature man and had no doubt seen many people with Parkinson's in his day. He was kind, gentle, and unhurried. We sensed that he was reluctant to tell us his diagnosis. At last, he told us that I was in the mild stages of Parkinson's disease and that it would take about ten years for me to enter the advanced stages. He advised me to go home, go back to work, and tell no one; no one would know. He told me nothing about medication, about what I would look and feel like in ten years, or about where I might get more information. And he did not explain why I should keep the diagnosis a secret.

Actually, we paid little attention to those mysteries at the moment. Blaine and I were too happy that the diagnosis was Parkinson's and not a brain tumor. At least Parkinson's wouldn't kill me. We wept with relief.

In the next weeks, I underwent CAT scans and other diagnostic tests to rule out other medical problems. At last my family doctor, who reviewed the tests, said that the results supported the neurologist's diagnosis. He agreed with the neurologist that I should exercise, keep up my good attitude, and keep on working. He, too, felt that I should tell no one and that no one need know.

I should have asked for more information, but my generation had been conditioned not to question the doctor; we'd learned to sit and agree to do what the doctor tells us to do. One thing I would have liked to know was why I shouldn't tell anyone. I realize that some patients really may not want to know any more than what the doctor tells them, but I was anxious to educate myself about this illness that had taken up residence in my body. I knew that it was progressive and that there was no cure. I knew a little about how the tremor acted, how one muscle worked against the other, how a person looked shuffling along all bent over. But that was all I knew.

I soon discovered that it would be difficult to educate myself: very little information was available, and I didn't know anyone else who had Parkinson's disease. Finally, Blaine learned of Merle Watson, a Parkinson's patient who lives in a neighboring town. I called Merle's wife, Barbara, and she gave me the addresses of the four national organizations concerned with Parkinson's disease. Their free materials, which I obtained in the mail, seemed to be the extent of the information available to patients in 1981. These depressing materials contained pictures of people with frozen facial expressions and thin, bent-over figures. Very little in the materials could give me much hope that I might live in reasonable comfort, as I later learned to live. However, I was now on several mailing lists, and soon newsletters began to appear. Within a year, more was being written, and what was written was more positive. (Although Parkinson's was not at the top of the researchers' lists when my disease was diagnosed, a renewed interest in Parkinson's generated much more research in subsequent years.)

By 1982, I knew I was going to retire from teaching. I had shared my "secret" of Parkinson's disease with my students and colleagues, as well as with my family and friends, and they were all very helpful. But it was not fair to have others do my work. Also, no matter how much they did, they could not take away the pain in my hips that made me limp, the all-over aching, and the extreme tiredness that kept me on the couch from the time I got home until bedtime.

It was frustrating that no one seemed to understand Parkinson's disease. The feeling kept growing in me that I needed to find an expert in the field. I learned the name of another neurologist, and in February 1982, I visited my second specialist. He, too, was helpful and understanding, and I certainly could not find any fault with him. But what I was really looking for was a specialist who lived and breathed Parkinson's disease. My family doctor and the neurologist had so many other illnesses to deal with. The question kept recurring in my mind: how much time do they really have to keep up with the latest findings on one disease—Parkinson's?

Finding my specialist in Parkinson's disease happened in a roundabout way. Blaine and I began thinking that we might start a Parkinson's support group in our area. We needed to talk to others with Parkinson's and felt that people in our area must have the same need. One person we talked to was Mary Dike of Gardiner, Maine, whom we contacted after reading about her in a newspaper article. Mary was also interested in starting a support group in her area. A home economics teacher a few years younger than I, Mary was about to leave teaching because of Parkinson's disease. She told us about her doctor, Robert Feldman, a Parkinson's specialist at Boston Medical Center. Listening to Mary, I felt that I had found the specialist I was looking for.

We made an appointment, and on April 2, 1983, I saw my third neurologist, Dr. Feldman. We were not disappointed. We found him and his multidisciplinary team to be experts whose aim was to educate the patient about Parkinson's disease and who knew how to treat the disease. They drew Blaine, me, and our family doctor into the "team." During that visit and at subsequent visits every six months, Dr. Feldman, Blaine, and I talked together until we agreed on a course of treatment that was satisfactory to all of us. Then Dr. Feldman wrote to our family doctor advising him of the results of our meeting. This is the pattern we still follow. Thus, I have the security of knowing that if I have any immediate problems, my family doctor, close by, knows my status.

I had come a long way since I first responded to my symptoms in 1980. I learned that I needed to take the responsibility of keeping myself as healthy as possible and to ask questions in the doctor's office. I learned that doctors, too, are human: some find it difficult to say, "I don't know," when they can't diagnose an illness. Some find it difficult to tell the patient when they do know. Some are insensitive. All doctors are different, just as all patients are different. It's important to find the right combination.

I feel that our persistence in looking for the right specialist has paid off. We feel good about our team.

Parkinson's is a progressive disease, but in most cases it progresses so slowly that it's easy to ignore the first symptoms. What are the first symptoms? They differ from person to person, but the ones I hear about most often are these:

- Fatigue
- Aches and pains that may be vague or may be severe enough to cause limping or all-over discomfort (they disappear when you rest for a while)
- Slow movement: this makes you feel like you are in a slow-motion segment of a movie or are walking through water
- Loss of the natural swing of your arms when you walk
- Poor balance and falling (a feeling of awkwardness)
- Tripping, caused by not lifting the feet sufficiently
- Dragging a foot
- Cramps or other weird sensations in the legs or the feet
- Difficulty with handwriting: sometimes you feel that each letter must be drawn painstakingly. The writing may get smaller and smaller as you progress, and sometimes the lines of your writing slant downhill. If you experience a tremor, your handwriting may be shaky.
- A jackknife effect when you touch your forefinger and middle finger together
- Difficulty with small objects requiring manual dexterity: buttoning clothes or fastening jewelry
- Symptoms that are more pronounced on one side of your body than on the other
- A vague feeling that something is not quite right

If you suspect that you have Parkinson's, knowing for certain will be much better than uncertainty. If your suspicions are confirmed, you can deal with your fears and find a Parkinson's specialist who will start you on a program of treatment. Educate yourself about the disease. Go to the library, write to the national organizations concerned with Parkinson's disease (see the names and addresses in the appendixes to this book), and join the nearest Parkinson's support group. Enlist the support, the confidence, and the involvement of your spouse, close relatives, or close friends from the beginning. You deserve the best!

CHAPTER 2

It's Not Fair!

God give us grace to accept with serenity
    The things that cannot be changed,
Courage to change the things
    That should be changed,
And the wisdom to distinguish the one
      from the other.
                —*Reinhold Niebuhr*, Serenity Prayer

The process of accepting and adjusting to life with Parkinson's disease probably began when I realized that the symptoms described in a newspaper's advice column matched my own. I became conscious of the process, though, after hearing the initial diagnosis by the first neurologist I saw. I would like to share some of that process with you. Let's back up to the end of that visit.

After Blaine and I learned that I had Parkinson's and left the first neurologist's office, we got into our car and started the four-hour drive back to our home in Maine. Those four hours were a special time for us. They belonged to us alone as we began the long journey of accepting Parkinson's into our busy lives. They were a time of preparation, a time of examining our feelings before we faced the questioning eyes of our children, our family, and our friends. The car was a haven where we had no interruptions.

Our first feelings were a mixture of relief and determination. We were relieved that the diagnosis was Parkinson's and not a brain tumor. We were determined that we could handle it. During periods of silence, we each contemplated what this meant to us. There were reassuring words. There were expressions of fear. There were tears at times, when the reality was too overwhelming. The most important message I received from Blaine came from the touch of his hand and from his attitude. No spoken words could have conveyed love and commitment as sincerely or as eloquently.

When we arrived home, we began to share what we had learned, first with our children, and then with our family and friends. We couldn't answer many of their questions because we knew so little ourselves. All we could do was accept their concern and reassure them that we could cope with the situation. We knew we could count on their support.

Eventually, I told my students. In spite of the fact that my doctor had said that no one would know, one of my students had already observed the difficulty I had in placing cookies on a plate and had laughed at it. I couldn't stand the thought of being laughed *at*. I preferred to have the students laugh *with* me. So one day I took advantage of an assignment that I had always used at the beginning of a new semester, which required each student to write a paper titled "Who Am I?" These papers, including my own paper, had always been shared aloud. In updating my paper, this time I concluded with information about my Parkinson's. I had found a rather painless way to share this news:

> I'm still all the things I was when I first wrote this paper, but I am more because of time. Changes take place that affect us.
>
> One wonderful change in my life is that I have become a grandmother. I have a granddaughter, Ashley, who lives next door, and a granddaughter, Bethany, who lives in Wisconsin. I'm sure you'll hear more about them as time goes by.

Another change in my life is harder to adjust to. I want to share it with you because it is a part of me, and if you accept me as a teacher and a friend, you have to accept me as I am. Last spring, I had to admit that something was happening to my body. Muscles in my right arm and leg were tight and feeling "lazy." I had difficulty writing, and I had a slight tremor in my right hand. I had become so slow moving, my family had begun to complain. A few students had made remarks that left me depressed. I suppose I was afraid to go to the doctor, but I finally did see several doctors. The diagnosis was Parkinson's disease. It's a progressive disease with no cure. However, there are medications that treat the symptoms, and a lot of research is being done now on Parkinson's. The best medicine in the beginning is good food, good exercise, and good attitude.

How is Parkinson's affecting me now? I have difficulty in moving and I tire easily. My coordination is not the best, and sometimes I lose my balance. But, so far, there's nothing I can't do that I did before—even if it takes a little longer. I'm determined to live a useful life, regardless of Parkinson's.

I think many people in our society go to great lengths to hide physical problems, as though they were something to be ashamed of. I don't want to do that. I think people—such as you, for instance—are capable of much understanding and compassion, but you can't understand me if I don't level with you. I'd rather laugh with you when I'm clumsy than have you laugh *at* me. I'm looking forward to this semester and getting to know you.

My students were wonderful. They were sympathetic, interested, and helpful. Several of them found the courage to talk to me about their own family members who were handicapped in some way.

In the world outside, when it seemed appropriate, I even told strangers. Sometimes when I fumbled for money at a checkout counter or held up some other line, I apologized for being so slow and explained that my Parkinson's was responsible. Many times, someone who overheard me would mention an acquaintance or a family member with Parkinson's and would ask questions. I found that talking about it helped me to accept it as a reality I could cope with. I was educating myself, and I didn't mind educating others, too, bit by bit.

In that early period, one of the things I found most difficult to deal with was waking up during the night and in the morning, having to face the fact that my Parkinson's was indeed a reality. Every day I worked at adjusting to it, but each new dawn meant starting all over. I tried various ways of making the realization less painful. Sometimes I planned one specific activity that I could look forward to on the following day; then I promised myself that I'd substitute the thought of that activity whenever my Parkinson's came to mind. Or I made up mental lists of things that I could still do that I could be thankful for. Try as I might, there seemed to be no way to prevent my mind from returning to my Parkinson's. I wish I could say that the emotional pain went away quickly, but it didn't. It was a very gradual process.

The first year or two, of course, were the worst. Anyone who has experienced great grief knows the feelings. First is a feeling of disbelief. Then there's the heavy, wretched feeling of "What am I going to do?" For a time, anger—the inescapable feeling that *it's not fair*—takes control.

Then, ever so slightly, the feelings ease. The long, constructive process of acceptance and adaptation begins in earnest.

Anger, an emotion I have always tended to hide, reappears from time to time. I've never been good at expressing it. I rarely raise my voice or complain, because I detest hearing others do so. I have trouble even admitting I *could* be angry. (Once when he was young, my son, Randy, mimicked family members for fun. When he imitated me, all of his body language and tone of voice showed anger, but he was forcing a wide smile and saying, "I'm not angry!" It was very funny—and an eye-opener for me.) In coming to terms with my Parkinson's, I needed to give myself permission to be angry at times, because the disease had upset my life. I had to learn to express a healthy amount of anger without feeling guilty about it.

I decided to try to deal openly with my anger in positive ways. I could go outdoors and walk it off. I could tackle the housework and allow myself to slam the cupboard doors. I could go to the typewriter and write about my feelings. What worked for me won't necessarily work for you, but the important thing is for you to admit that you have normal emotions, look at how you deal with them, and allow yourself not to feel guilty about having them.

I bring up the subject of guilt because you may have grown up hearing the same homespun wisdom that I heard: "Well, your problem could be a lot worse" and "What if you had what Jane Smith has?" It's true that there are always people in worse circumstances than our own, but knowing of their conditions doesn't lessen our pain. Each person has a right to his or her share of sympathy and understanding, according to need. We don't have to feel guilty because we become angry or need a shoulder to cry on. Problems arise only when we prolong the complaints, which prevents us from ultimately picking ourselves up and getting on with life.

Over the years, one of the hardest things for me to control has been worry. Worry, of course, uses a lot of energy. It is unproductive and useless. Despite these disincentives, I have to admit that I still do some worrying. Fortunately, in my set of mixed feelings, the balance is more positive than negative. I fear what is ahead, but I immediately think of the current, ongoing research that will provide me with more protection. I resent all the limitations, but at the same time, I'm so thankful for all the things I can still do.

Since 1981, I've lived with the knowledge that I have Parkinson's. I still pray each day for a cure, but the feelings of misery are gone. Although I still grumble when I get up at night and find myself shuffling along, I have other things to think about when I wake up in the morning. Does this mean that I have totally accepted and adjusted to the fact that I have Parkinson's? No, it doesn't. I know that accepting and adjusting are continual processes. But I can see that I'm doing a reasonably good job of adjusting and accepting. I don't like Parkinson's, but I've got it, and I've proved to myself that I can handle it and still lead a productive life.

As time has gone by, my frustrations have changed as my Parkinson's has changed. Some things in life have become more difficult, but I haven't given up. Now when I have a "freezing" or a dizzy spell, I know that in a few minutes it will pass. I still try to do as many things as I did in the past, but I have to make allowances.

Life goes on—you can go with it or stop living.

As with most things, it seems that with Parkinson's, what goes around comes around. Even when I felt somewhat energetic and capable, I still noticed little, sneaky symptoms cropping up, like the incident with the plate of cookies. Then when I lost hope and was almost ready to give up, things improved and I started the cycle all over again. Life gets harder in one way, but it seems to make up for this in other ways. I haven't given up yet, and I consider myself fortunate that I've had very little tremor.

CHAPTER 3

Coping with Frustration: Practical Suggestions for Everyday Living

If my brain can conceive it,
And my mind can believe it,
Then I can achieve it.

—*Anonymous*

Parkinson's disease interferes to some degree with all the bodily movements that people take for granted. The most ordinary tasks and activities become difficult and taxing, especially toward the end of a dose of medication. This interference in everyday activities produces deep feelings of frustration in the person with Parkinson's—feelings that I, for one, have never been able to overcome entirely. However, I have found ways to minimize the problems that cause these feelings, and they are worth sharing with you. I hope that they will help you, as well, to live a full and interesting life.

At the outset, you should know that current medications and therapies enable people with Parkinson's to have a normal life and live it more comfortably than ever before. While there is no way to eliminate all the frustrations you will experience with Parkinson's disease, there is a positive approach to coping, if you will make that choice.

My own earliest frustrations began with the onset of my symptoms. On the right side of my body, where my symptoms had started, I moved where I wasn't supposed to move and didn't move where I expected to move. In addition, I experienced strange, unexplained sensations in my right arm and leg.

Later, the keys to our home and car "didn't work" for me, although they still worked for Blaine. The window shades wouldn't roll up. Jar lids wouldn't come off or go back on. Manufacturers seemed as if they were out to get me, with bottles covered by child-proof caps, cereal boxes and dry goods sealed with unyielding glue, and other containers double-locked with tough, extra packaging seals. I knew that all of these closures were designed for added safety, but, oh! The frustration!

To make matters worse, I began to trip on steps and curbs that I could see perfectly clearly. My hand shook a little, so that finer skills, such as writing, became difficult. My walk slowed, and my right arm no longer swung normally. I became stiff and achy. And why, I wondered, was I so tired all of the time? I knew that if I were to cope with these new problems, I would have to understand more about what was happening to me.

After we found Dr. Feldman and the Parkinson's Program at Boston Medical Center and learned more about Parkinson's disease, I understood better. In Parkinson's, the level of natural dopamine in the brain is low. *Dopamine* is a substance produced by the body that is necessary for carrying messages within the brain. A lowered level of dopamine ultimately permits too many muscles to contract at once. One muscle starts pushing hard against another, each muscle canceling the action of the other, and this abnormal pushing of muscle against muscle is very fatiguing. One has to work much harder to complete a movement. Also, because of the resistance, movement is slowed down. Why was I so tired? My body was exhausting itself by trying to compensate for the changes taking place and by fighting the abnormal movements.

Armed with this knowledge, Blaine and I solved one of my early problems: tripping. Blaine had started to watch me very closely, and he noticed that my right foot was always the one that tripped. We theorized that over my lifetime, I had probably programmed my brain to tell me how to react to a step or a curb. Thus, the brain got the message that a small rise was in my way, and it sent a message to lift my foot a certain amount. Now, however, with muscle pushing against muscle, the brain didn't raise my foot as high with the same amount of energy it had used for years, so I tripped. We decided that I had to retrain and reprogram my brain. I would have to be very specific at first. When I saw a step or a curb, I would have to tell my brain to call for a little more lift from my right leg. I put my mind to this, and the reprogramming worked: the tripping stopped. In the years since, tripping has caused me only two falls, both times because I was running in bad weather.

Soon I applied the same retraining to other everyday tasks. I reprogrammed my brain to make me turn the key harder, exert more energy to open jars and boxes, and forcefully pull up the window shades. Although I felt weak at times, I knew that my muscles were strong and would remain strong, unless I stopped using and exercising them. Even when I felt so weak that I could hardly move, I knew that when my brain got a supply of dopamine, my muscles would be ready to go to work again.

During my first years with Parkinson's, before I began taking medication, difficulty with writing was an especially frustrating problem, because teaching requires so much writing. My colleagues in the home economics department volunteered to do much of my writing, and they had a stamp made of my signature, so that I wouldn't have to sign so many student passes and papers. People with Parkinson's can manage a typewriter better than a pen, so I started using a typewriter. Interestingly, I found that I could still write on the chalkboard, because the larger muscles are used in that activity.

As time went by, I felt that I was imposing more and more on my colleagues. It was not fair that they should have to do my work as well as their own.

During this time period, I began to feel twinges of pain in my hips, which I theorized were the result of my right side being out of sync with my left. Soon the twinges turned to stiffness and pain. I began to limp. As long as I got a good night's sleep, I felt well in the morning, but by noon I really had to push myself. When I came home from school in the afternoon, I was so tired that I often flopped on the couch and remained there. By 1982, I was not sleeping well. Overtired and achy, I tossed and turned and talked in my sleep—and kept Blaine from sleeping, too. The stress of pushing myself to perform the way I had always performed took a mental and physical toll on me and left me too tired to think. We decided that teaching, which is a challenge even for a healthy person, had become too much for me. Retiring, after twenty-six full years of teaching, was the right thing to do.

After retirement, things changed for me. I felt much better because I could pace myself and take frequent rests. But because I was not yet taking medication, my frustrating problems with aches and tiredness still kept me from doing housework and inviting guests for dinner.

The answer to these early postretirement problems came when we consulted Dr. Feldman in 1982. With the decision that I would start medication, one-half of the lowest-dosage Sinemet pill in the morning and the other half at noon, came the relief of many of my symptoms—and hope for the future. (In chapter 8 you can learn more about Sinemet and other medications.)

Here I want to suggest that if your Parkinson's symptoms are seriously affecting your quality of living, there are two important areas to consider: medication and lifestyle. First evaluate your medication with your doctor. Then take a good look at your lifestyle. Ask yourself: Is my job too demanding now? Am I carrying too many responsibilities in the organizations to which I belong? Am I getting enough household help? Do I have opportunities to rest during the day? Do I get enough sleep? Am I sitting in front of the television too much of the time and not getting enough exercise? Am I alone too much?

Answer the questions honestly and be willing to make changes. Early retirement, for example, is not the end of the world. It can open doors to a whole new life. Learn to pace yourself. No one else can do it for you. Help yourself, but learn to accept help from people around you. Try new activities. You may surprise yourself! I played miniature golf recently and did better than Blaine. At a friend's wedding last year I danced with Blaine and rediscovered a love of dancing—despite my conviction that I would never be able to dance again! Exercise every day. Involve yourself in one or two clubs or organizations that keep you in touch with people. Get a dog or a cat to keep you company at home.

To make life easier, you can modify your home environment. We have found that changes we made in the bedroom and the bathroom were very helpful. For example, we recommend the king-size, baffled water bed that we bought. (The water is contained in several separate tubes or chambers so that the mattress remains motionless.) I disturb Blaine less when I move around on this big bed, and I move around less because I am more comfortable on a bed that accommodates the contours of the body so well. Water beds come with adjustable temperature settings; the warmth of the bed alleviates the pain in my hips and adds comfort not only for me but also for Blaine, who has some arthritis. Satin sheets and satin nightwear make moving around in bed easier.

Because exercise is important to people with Parkinson's, Blaine moved my stationary bicycle and my rowing machine into the bedroom where they would be more convenient for me. He relocated a wall in our bedroom to create room for the machines.

During the remodeling of the adjoining bathroom, Blaine installed an extra-large, square, bathtub-shower combination, in which two corners of the tub contain built-in seats. I can bathe more safely when I am seated. At the sides of the tub, he installed two grab-bars for extra protection. He also installed a high-rise toilet made for handicapped people, which is easier to rise from than a regular toilet. However, you don't have to remodel your bathroom to obtain some of these safety features. A waterproof, adjustable tub seat and a portable, over-the-toilet commode with armrests can be purchased at the nearest medical/surgical supply store. A grab-bar that clamps onto the tub or a wall bar can also be purchased. These items are well worth the expense.

It makes sense to go through your home carefully, to see what changes can be made for comfort and safety. Railings need to be installed on stairways and grab-bars beside all steps. A grab-bar can be installed on the wall beside your bed, too. Or, if your bed is the standard type (with a mattress and a box spring), you can clamp on a device called Helping Handle anywhere along the side of the bed; it will give you a handhold to help you pull yourself up. This device can be slipped off and taken with you when you travel. (For information about Helping Handle, call Maxi-Aids Inc.'s toll-free number 800-522-6294, or write to them at 42 Executive Boulevard, Farmingdale, NY 11735.) Another handhold could be a knotted rope, one end of which is tied to the bed frame at the foot of the bed. The other end lies on top of the covers where you can reach it easily and pull yourself up. An aid to help you shift your position in bed is a trapeze. This is a bar bent into a triangle, suspended from a metal arm; the arm is clamped onto the head of the bed.

Some people with Parkinson's find that they can move around more easily on a bed with a very firm mattress. Others place a chair with armrests in the bedroom, so that they can sit comfortably while they dress.

In the bathroom, you may want to use an electric razor instead of a blade. (If you need to, you can move your face across the razor, instead of the razor across your face.) If you find your toothbrush difficult to manipulate, use an electric toothbrush and a Water Pik oral hygiene device. Or you may want to try an instrument called Interplak, which acts as both a toothbrush and a flosser. Some people with Parkinson's find that they can manage a regular toothbrush more easily if they put a large, foam-rubber hair curler or a rubber bicycle handle grip over the handle of the brush. In the bathroom, unbreakable plastic or paper cups are safer than glass or ceramic.

If you experience difficulty in bathing with your washcloth, try using a terrycloth mitt, a long-handled brush, or a sponge. When soap falls to the floor of the tub, it creates a slippery hazard. Hanging soap-on-a-rope on a faucet will keep the soap from getting too far away from you. To prevent slipping in the wet tub, wear mesh, rubber-soled shoes when you bathe, and use a rubber mat on the floor of the tub or the shower stall when you shower. Instead of a small, loose bath rug outside your tub or shower stall, prevent tripping by installing wall-to-wall carpet in the bathroom.

Are you aware of all the special equipment for home use that is available at your nearest medical supply store? Ask the salesperson to show you equipment that's useful for people with Parkinson's. Did you know that some major department stores also have catalogs with special aids and special clothing? (See appendix D for many sources of special equipment and clothing.)

Do you have a telephone beside your bed? That's an important place to have one. If you have difficulty speaking loudly enough, you may want to obtain a device from the telephone company that will amplify your telephone voice. (For the AT&T Special Needs number nearest you, call 800-555-1212.) Another convenience is a speakerphone, which you do not have to hold; it leaves your hands free. Cordless phones are helpful because they have no wires to trip over. Another useful appliance in the bedroom is a radio or a cassette player that can be set to turn itself off: soothing music will help you fall asleep.

Has your hearing been affected? You can get an amplifier for your telephone and a closed-caption device for your television set.

Housekeeping chores can be very frustrating for someone with Parkinson's. You can help yourself by using a small, rolling cart to carry cleansers, implements, and other items through the house. Another cart can carry food from the kitchen to the dining area. An apron with large pockets is also useful for carrying items back to their proper places when you tidy up. If you use a walker, you can attach a bicycle basket to it to carry items in the house.

When you prepare a meal, cook double or triple the amount of food, and freeze the extra portions for future meals. Cook several items side by side in the same steamer pot—you'll have fewer pots to wash. Even leftovers or frozen, precooked foods can be added next to items that are already steaming. An electric can opener makes opening cans much easier. A nutcracker can be used to unscrew the lids of small jars. (Special lid openers are also available for this purpose.) If you keep a sponge mop handy in the kitchen, you can wipe up spills as soon as they occur.

Bed making will be easier if you use a comforter that doubles as a spread. To write shopping lists, notes, and letters, try using a clipboard to keep the paper steady. A felt-tip pen may be easier to write with than other pens are. If you notice that your handwriting decreases rapidly in size (a common problem among people with Parkinson's), try this trick: stop writing, pick up your arm, wiggle your fingers, and start writing again. Use wide-lined paper to guide your writing.

Is grocery shopping a hassle for you? You may want to shop during off-hours—early in the morning, for example—to avoid crowds and lines.

Have you checked to see if you qualify for Meals on Wheels?

Just as there are many ways to make life easier in the home, you can also reduce frustration in the car. First you must ask

yourself, can you continue to drive? Before I started taking medication, I noticed (after learning how to make the key open the
car door) that I was taking longer to make turns. I saw that I wasn't
moving the steering wheel as far as before. Several times my foot
felt stuck to the gas pedal. I couldn't exert enough pressure on the
seat adjustment lever while pulling up at the same time, to move
the seat to a comfortable position for driving. I thought, "This is
it!" The possibility of not being able to drive was frightening.
Fortunately, after I started taking medication, I was able to drive
safely, but I have put restrictions on myself. I don't drive long dis-
tances because doing so causes my muscles to tighten up and hurt.
I also don't drive if I don't feel well, the weather is bad, or the
roads are icy.

Now I can adjust the car seat easily because our new car has
power seat adjustments, a very good option for people with Parkinson's. By having the car serviced regularly and having good
tires on the car at all times, we minimize the chance of car trouble
when I am out alone. And I always keep an extra supply of medication in the glove compartment, just in case I forget to put it in
my purse. (Be sure to discard unused medications at the end of
each summer, because heat makes them unstable.)

Getting in and out of a car can be difficult for people who
have Parkinson's. I like to make my own way, but I don't object if
someone extends a steadying hand. A satin cloth fastened down
on the seat makes sliding in and out much easier. Some people
use a large plastic bag tucked into the seat. Beaded seat cushions
also work very well.

Are you a passenger who needs another person's help to get
out of the car? Wide canvas belts are available in medical supply
stores, which can be put around your waist to give your caregiver
something to hold and pull while assisting you out of the car. You
should always sit in the front seat; the back seat is much more difficult to get out of.

If walking from the car to the store is difficult, you can obtain
special license plates for the handicapped that permit you to park

in designated areas nearest the store. (You don't have to be the driver of the car to obtain these special plates.)

When you go out for a drive, you can avoid problems by carrying extra medication and a plastic water bottle or a thermos of water for taking pills.

As a person with Parkinson's, you experience many frustrating difficulties in the course of each day. Fortunately, there are ways to cope and minimize their effect on your life. One of the most serious difficulties is the tendency to fall. Ordinarily, when people begin to tip or lose their balance, their bodies make some automatic adjustments, and they catch themselves. However, by the time someone with Parkinson's has made the adjustments, the person may already be down.

If you have experienced the problem of falling, what should you do? First, try to remember when, where, and why you fell. Then determine what you can do to avoid those circumstances in the future, and train yourself to practice preventive measures. For example, if you notice that you fall when you open the refrigerator door, you may need to change the way you open it. Don't stand in front of the door because you will have to step back, and people with Parkinson's fall backward very easily. Stand to one side and then open the door. When we replaced our old refrigerator, we bought a side-by-side model. The doors are not as wide, and they work great.

Do you lose your balance when you open doors to rooms and hallways? Ordinary handles can be installed on walls near doorknobs so that you can hold onto the handle with one hand and turn the doorknob with the other. This arrangement will help to keep you steady while you open a door. If you have trouble with doorknobs, you can purchase rubberlike lever handles from a health supply outlet to fit over the doorknobs. Or, you can replace the knobs themselves with lever-type handles.

To prevent tripping and slipping, remove doorsills, scatter rugs, footstools, and other impediments, and forget about waxing floors. Avoid wearing shoes with rubber or crepe soles; they catch and stick to the floor. Be sure to put night-lights in the bathroom and the hallways, as well as beside any steps; night-lights are a must for people with Parkinson's.

In walking and standing, you can help to prevent falls by keeping your feet about eight inches apart; this stance widens your base of support. If you have a tendency to retropulse (to walk backward), then always keep one foot back when you stand still. When you walk, keep your body upright and as tall as possible: if your upper body is leaning forward (as is frequently the case with people who have Parkinson's), you will fall more easily. A trick that dancers use to help them stand tall is to imagine that they are suspended from the ceiling (or the sky) by an elastic string attached to the top of the head; the elastic string exerts a gentle pull upward. See if it works for you.

Do not hurry when you walk. Some people with Parkinson's have a tendency to speed up as they move along, until they can no longer control their speed and balance. You may want to stop frequently and start again slowly.

Use a cane if it will help you to keep your balance. Some people with Parkinson's like to use a walking stick, rather than a cane, because the stick helps them to stand up straighter. In stores, take advantage of the shopping cart: it frees you from having to carry items and using one steadies your walk. Some people with Parkinson's use walkers, but a walker that you have to lift and walk with is not suited to everyone because of the many different movements that it requires at one time. A walker with wheels mounted under the legs is useful for some people. The walker should have brakes on the handles so that it won't roll out of control.

When you walk, you can free your hands by carrying your money, keys, medication, and identification in a fanny pack strapped around your waist; you don't have to carry a handbag. Some people sew large pockets with Velcro closures onto their clothes and on the insides of their coats to hold their personal items. This may be another way to free your hands from handbags.

Because of balance and coordination problems, people with Parkinson's tend to fall when they make turns. When you turn, make a U-turn (walk in the pattern of the letter U), instead of pivoting in place.

Still another cause of falling is the muscular condition known as "freezing." Freezing reminds me of the childhood game Statues, in which we danced about until the leader called "Freeze!" and we froze in whatever position we were in at that moment. For some reason, people with Parkinson's often "freeze" when they approach a doorway, a doorsill, a scatter rug, a step, or a curb, but others freeze when they are merely walking along or crossing a street.

To break the freeze, you must use a little trick to get yourself moving again before you lose your balance and fall. Some people are able to break a freeze by imagining a line or a small object on the floor and stepping over it. Others imagine that they are marching, and this enables them to go ahead. Some are able to rock back and forth and then go on. Still others do it by lifting one foot and kicking the other foot with it. Sometimes a distraction will break the freeze. Try counting, aloud or silently. Try moving sideways instead of forward. If someone is present, ask for a hand.

To deal with rising from a fall, it may be a good idea to practice getting down onto the floor and getting yourself up, once a day. If you can't seem to get up, crawl over to the nearest stable object or railing and pull yourself up. (Be sure to do this practice only in the presence of another person who can help you.)

Always wear a Medic-Alert bracelet. I always wear mine. In case I fall or am involved in an accident, I want the hospital or any doctor to know about my medication needs. It may also be a good idea to keep a list of your medications, the doses, and any allergies to medications in your purse or wallet and on your wall (where it can be easily seen) at home. Be sure to update these lists whenever there are changes. Another good idea is to keep a list of important telephone numbers in your wallet and another copy displayed on the wall near your telephone: doctor, hospital, ambulance, caregivers, close family members, fire department, and police. In an emergency, neighbors or rescue squad members will see the list and know whom to call.

Many people with Parkinson's experience frequent dizziness, light-headedness, and occasional fainting. I have that problem, particularly on hot, humid days or in poorly ventilated rooms. It also happens when I get out of bed in the morning or get up from a chair. I've found that wearing elastic stockings is helpful in stuffy rooms or humid weather. Before I get up from a seated position, I wiggle my feet to get the blood circulating.

When I am away from home, I always check the surrounding area to see where I could sit down quickly if I needed to, and I try to avoid poorly ventilated places. If I feel faint, I sit down or lie down. If I see no place to sit, I try to keep moving to keep my blood circulating, because the faintness is worst when I stand still.

My first experience with fainting came when I had a bad cramp in my leg, and, without thinking, I jumped out of bed to stand on it. Instead, I became dizzy and had only enough time to sit on the bed before I fainted. Luckily, Blaine woke up and found me. I resolved then to avoid any other fast starts. Now, when I get up, I do it in stages: first, I sit on the edge of the bed for a while, then I stand up.

Getting up from a bed or a chair is an automatic movement for most people, but it can be an exercise in frustration for the person with Parkinson's. Although special lift chairs are available for people in the advanced stages of Parkinson's, you should probably avoid them for as long as possible, because they deprive you of much-needed exercise. If your chair is a solid one, slide forward to the front edge of the seat, rock back and forth, and, on the count of three, stand up. (Sometimes I fall back into the seat and have to start over. If someone takes my hand, that seems to get me going.) If the chair is a puffy, soft, easy chair, place your hands firmly on each side of the seat or on each arm and raise yourself. Although you may feel weak, your muscles are still strong and they will work for you. (As Dr. Feldman told us, a person with

Parkinson's can feel so feeble that he believes he can't get out of a chair, but if someone were to yell "Fire!" he'd be the first one out of the door!)

Another source of frustration for people with Parkinson's may be impediments to eating—one of life's special pleasures! But eating can still be enjoyable if you are willing to make a few adjustments. One of the most important ones is arranging to take your dose of Sinemet about three-quarters of an hour to an hour before mealtime, rather than at the meal. Taking your medication before the meal will make it likely that your medication is working when you start the meal. (If you have difficulty splitting and swallowing your pills, there are pill splitters and special glasses that make swallowing pills easier. If your medications make your mouth dry, try moistening your mouth with a sip of water beforehand and take your pill with a bit of Jell-O or applesauce.)

You can also make other adjustments. Chew and swallow slowly; hurrying increases the possibility of choking. (If you have difficulty swallowing properly, a speech therapist can teach you how to swallow safely.) Must you eat steak? You may want to ask someone to cut it up for you. Break spaghetti into small pieces. (Spaghetti is a food I enjoy at home but avoid in restaurants.) A plastic apron prevents food spills from staining your clothes. If your food or drinks have a way of getting away from you, you may want to stock your kitchen with the special silverware, dishes, and glasses that are sold in medical supply stores. Utensils with especially wide handles and spill-proof cups may make your life easier. Ordinary flexible straws, available in the supermarket, also help with drinking, especially if the cup is only partially full. A plate guard that encircles your plate keeps food from being shoved off the edge and provides a place to push food onto your fork. (A wide soup bowl or a serving bowl may serve the same purpose.) Plates and cups can be set on rubber mats to keep them from sliding off the table.

What foods can you comfortably order at a restaurant? Keep them in mind when you eat out, so that you will not have to worry about how you will get the food to your mouth. If you have special forks and so forth at home, bring them with you to the restaurant. Some people with Parkinson's cannot manage tasks that require using both hands, such as cutting food. If you have this difficulty, ask the server to bring your food already cut up.

When I eat out, I take along a damp handkerchief in a plastic sandwich bag to sponge any spots that may result from spilling or dropping a bit of food. Small wipes, in individual packets, are also easy to carry in your purse or leave in your car.

If you find it difficult to get food to your mouth because of a pronounced tremor or involuntary movements of the arm and the hand, try strapping one-pound weights (with Velcro closures) onto your wrists. They will steady your hands as you carry food to your mouth, and at the same time, they will help build up strength in your arm muscles. (See more about eating in chapter 4.)

A source of frustration to most people with Parkinson's is the difficulty they experience in dressing and undressing. One woman told me that she has seen her husband take five minutes just to remove his hat. Another source of frustration is the irritation that some caregivers express when people with Parkinson's can dress or shave themselves on some days, but not on others. They say, "If you can do it now, you can do it any time. Sometimes you just don't try." What you must convey to the caregiver is that your medication does a good job when it is working, but sometimes it wears off and then you have to wait for the next surge.

Whenever you are able to dress without help, you should take your time to do so, because the movements involved in dressing provide valuable exercise. If the caregiver becomes impatient with the pace, he or she should leave the room. However, some clothing can be too difficult to cope with, without aid. (Have you ever gotten something over your head, with one arm in, and the other partially in, and been stuck there? That's when you need help!) To make life easier, give away any clothes that are too tight or have too many buttons. For clothes with very few buttons, buy a special button-hooking device, or try pushing a paper clip through the buttonhole, catching the button, and pulling it back out the buttonhole.

What kind of clothes do you need? Clothes that are loose enough to be comfortable. Clothes that have Velcro closures. Even shoes with Velcro closures are available. At a support group meeting, one of the participants, Barbara, told us about the time she left her husband, Merle, to dress himself and later found that he had cut his shoelaces because he had become so frustrated with trying to tie them! Merle would probably appreciate shoes with Velcro closures, slip-on shoes, or elasticized laces that always remain tied. An extra-long shoehorn is helpful for getting shoes on. Tube socks (straight socks without toe and heel contours) are easier to put on than regular socks, and they are just as comfortable. Because Parkinson's affects the small muscles of the toes, don't wear backless shoes; your toes may not keep them on properly.

When selecting clothing that is comfortable and easy to put on, don't neglect style and appearance. You want attractive clothing, and if you are a woman, you'll want to continue using cosmetics. If you are well groomed and attractively dressed, you'll feel better about yourself, and you'll walk a little taller.

Speech problems, up to and including the loss of one's voice, are fearful prospects, but they are frustrating realities for some people with Parkinson's. When I was a child, I had a great deal I wanted to say, but I was too shy to say it. Gradually, I overcame my shyness and discovered the joy of speaking. The possibility of losing my voice to Parkinson's was very upsetting, but so far, it has not happened. Exercising the vocal cords is very important. I do it often, especially when I'm alone in the car, driving down the highway; I turn the radio on and sing along as loudly as I please. I also do my part in leading the discussion in the support group and speak whenever I'm asked.

If you have a problem with your speech, such as a low, flat tone or a mumble, find a speech therapist who can teach you the correct exercises to help you preserve your voice. Do it without delay as soon as you realize that you have a problem. Make a habit of using the phone each day; you will exercise your voice while you keep in touch with your family and friends. Sing, recite poetry, and talk to your pet. Above all, don't let your spouse or caregiver speak for you.

The unusual movements that people with Parkinson's sometimes experience are another source of frustration. If this happens to you, talk with your doctor. Be aware that the tremor of Parkinson's is a fine shake that stops when you start to reach for something. Larger, spasmodic movements of the arms and the hands or twisting movements of the feet, the legs, or even the whole body (called "dyskinesias") are probably toxic effects of overmedication. If you begin to have this kind of problem, you should call your doctor. You may need a change in your medication or even a drug holiday. (See chapter 8 for more about toxic reactions, side effects, and drug holidays.)

Another frustrating side effect of overmedication may be hallucinations. If you experience hallucinations, tell your doctor immediately, so that he or she can modify your medications or get you situated for a drug holiday. While hallucinating, a person finds it very difficult, of course, to distinguish between what is real and what is not. Our friend Merle hallucinates and has been generous enough to share his experiences with our support group. He has a wonderful sense of humor and sees the funny side of the ordeal of hallucinating, though he admits that it is also very disturbing. He has found that the best way for him to distinguish between real and unreal people is to reach out to touch them. The unreal people "disappear." He asked Barbara to tell our group about one incredible incident, which he calls his "fiasco," because he knew we would appreciate the comedy while we learned how serious hallucinations can be.

One night, Merle awoke to "see" a man with a cigarette going through a bureau. Merle is a man in the advanced stages of Parkinson's who needs help getting out of a chair and who walks with great difficulty. Believing that he was being burglarized, however, he managed to get out of his special hospital-style bed to telephone the police. Holding the phone upside down in his haste, he thought the phone didn't work because the "burglar" had cut the wires. Because he was unable to use the phone, he raised the window (luckily, on the ground floor), crawled out, and let himself down to his huge, terraced lawn. He rolled down three lawns and over to the next house, where he asked the neighbors to call the police. When the police arrived, they found everything intact and Barbara still asleep!

Sharing this experience with the group made it less formidable for Merle, just as relating our experiences has helped each of us to adjust to them. You, too, can help yourself and others by sharing your feelings and frustrations in a support group. It's good to find other people who experience what you are going through, so that, together, you can find ways to cope. (See more about support groups in chapter 14.)

There has been a great deal of material in this chapter for you to digest, about coping with the frustrations of daily living that are common to people with Parkinson's. You may want to reread this chapter before going on to the next topic, "Nutrition That Affects Our Lives."

CHAPTER 4

Nutrition That Affects Our Lives

Thy food shall be thy remedy.

—Hippocrates

If we are really serious about controlling our Parkinson's symptoms, we are very deliberate about eating well. Our level of nutrition affects the quality of our lives.

For some of us, balancing a diet and meeting our special needs may be a bit tricky without proper management. In this chapter, I want to share with you the aspects of nutrition that are unique to people with Parkinson's and some techniques for assuring that our bodies get what they really need.

The first thing we have to remember is how important it is to maintain a body weight that is appropriate for our size and build. Your doctor should determine the optimum weight for you to maintain, but until you get his or her recommendation, you can use this method of calculation: for women, start with 100 pounds and add 5 pounds for every inch over 5 feet; for men, start with 106 pounds and add 6 pounds for every inch over 5 feet. Adjust the total down a bit if you have a very narrow build and up a bit if you have a wide build.

Ask your doctor or dietitian to tell you the total daily caloric intake that will maintain your appropriate weight. Pin up a calorie chart and become familiar with the caloric values of the foods you eat. Most high-protein foods are also high-calorie foods. (Proteins also contain important amino acids, which our bodies use in many ways.) Four portions of high-protein foods are recommended each day: generally, two portions from the meat-poultry-fish-and-eggs group of foods, and two portions from the milk-and-cheese group. Many people with Parkinson's lose more weight than they should, which depletes their bodies of protein and muscle, along with fat. They can't afford that because body protein and muscle are absolutely necessary, not only for strength and endurance but also for responding to physical and emotional stress.

People with Parkinson's tend to lose weight because of a number of problems. Some people have frequent tremors, which use up energy. Tremors also complicate getting food to the mouth, which discourages eating. Others have difficulty with cutting up food and give up in embarrassment or frustration. Some people find it hard to chew or swallow foods. Some have a sluggish digestive system and a feeling of fullness that keeps them from eating when mealtime comes. Yet others are simply depressed.

You can overcome a number of obstacles to eating by taking your Sinemet three-quarters of an hour or an hour before you eat. (Observe the length of time that's necessary for your pill to start working, and schedule your medication for that amount of time before the meal). Typically, people who take their Sinemet pill at mealtime are at the end of their last dose. By the time they get help from the new dose, they are finished with their meal. They have lost their appetite because of the struggle to get food to their mouths, chew, and swallow. But someone who takes the pill forty-five to sixty minutes before eating can have a more successful and enjoyable meal because the medication is already working.

Taking the first dose in the morning, almost an hour before breakfast, may present a problem at first. I remember the first morning I took my Sinemet that way and experienced "morning sickness," although I knew I wasn't pregnant. My doctor suggested that I take the early morning pill with milk, which I did. I found that milk eliminated the nausea. Once my body adapted to the medication, I was able to take the pill without milk or food of any kind. (Now scientists know that protein interferes with Sinemet, and they advise taking that early morning pill with a dry cracker or toast instead of milk.) Studies show that more benefit is derived from the Sinemet if it is taken on an empty stomach. It can be absorbed into the bloodstream immediately and can travel to the brain to start working. If it is taken with food, it has to compete with everything else that is eaten, and some of the effectiveness is lost. (Unfortunately, some Sinemet still comes from pharmacies with instructions that it be taken with food. Often, I talk with people who, mistakenly, think they *have* to take it with food. You may wish to discuss this point with your doctor.)

If you take your medication at the appropriate time but are still troubled by tremorous hands during eating, you may want to ask your doctor for an additional medication to control tremor. Or you may want to try strapping small, one-pound weights with Velcro closures onto your wrists while you eat; they help in controlling tremor. These weights can be found in a medical/surgical supply store or can be ordered through your local pharmacy or hospital.

If, despite medication, you still have difficulty cutting up your food, you may want to ask someone to do it for you before you sit down to eat. Or you could invest in an electric food processor to help with the task. The food processor is a good investment because it can also help you become a creative cook, preparing many tasty mixtures of foods.

If you have a dry mouth (caused by certain medications) or have difficulty chewing or swallowing, you can also use the food processor or, to a lesser extent, a blender to mix your food with liquid and chop or puree it. Eat slowly and deliberately. Give yourself time to eat your whole meal. Of course, if you have difficulty swallowing, you should ask your doctor to refer you to a therapist (usually, a speech therapist) who can teach you how to think through the steps of swallowing and enable you to eat your meal safely. Swallowing food improperly may cause food particles to travel into your lungs, where any foreign matter can cause pneumonia. You don't need that! Most people with swallowing difficulties know that liquid is even more difficult to swallow correctly than is pureed or well-chewed food. It seems to be harder for the muscles to direct liquid along the right pathway, and liquid that makes its way into the lungs can also cause pneumonia. The speech therapist will teach you how to swallow liquids correctly.

In the booklet *Speech Problems and Swallowing Problems in Parkinson's Disease*, the American Parkinson Disease Association offers the following suggestions for dealing with eating difficulties:

> Before you actually start eating, think through the steps of swallowing: lips closed, teeth together, food on the tongue, lift the tongue up—then back and swallow. (UP-BACK-SWALLOW.)
>
> Prevent the problem of food buildup by eating slowly and taking small amounts at a time. Swallow small, well-chewed morsels only.
>
> Chew your food hard, and move the food around with your tongue. Make an effort to chew first on one side, then the other.
>
> Don't put additional food in your mouth until you have swallowed the previous mouthful.
>
> Ask your family and other caring persons to learn the Heimlich maneuver in the event you suffer a choking episode. A physician or other health professional can explain the procedure.

Because people with Parkinson's slow down inside as well as outside, a common problem is constipation. Sometimes the constipation is caused by medications. With constipation comes a loss of the desire to eat, as well as gas buildup, headache, and increased rigidity and tremor. In order to combat constipation, people with Parkinson's need a great deal of liquid. You should drink at least eight to ten glasses of liquid a day, including water, fruit juices (especially prune and grape juice), bouillon, coffee, tea, and other soft drinks. The extra liquid helps to keep things moving along as they should.

To combat constipation, the Parkinson's diet must also include many high-fiber foods to add bulk, such as fresh and dried fruits, garden salads, cooked vegetables, legumes, brown rice, barley, pasta, bran and bran cereals, and whole-grain bread. The added bulk helps to keep things moving. Be sure to keep a covered dish of stewed fruit in the refrigerator: select a mixture of dried prunes, mixed dried fruits, and raisins or dried apricots; put them in a medium saucepan; sprinkle with a bit of ground cinnamon; add just enough water to cover the fruit; and cook for a few minutes until the fruit is soft. Yum! You can spoon out a little with any meal or make a snack of them. Alongside the stewed fruit, keep a bowl of cut-up raw veggies to dip into anytime. You can have salad at every lunch and dinner. Be creative about cooking your vegetables. In a small steamer pot, you can steam tasty medleys of several types of vegetables, including a small onion for flavor. When they are done, transfer them to a bowl and toss them either with a bit of olive oil and basil or oregano or with butter and salt.

Add split-pea soup, kidney beans, chickpeas, brown rice, and barley to your lunches and dinners. Cook enough for several meals, and store the leftovers in a covered bowl in the refrigerator. A portion can be taken out and rewarmed in a steamer pot (along with leftover meat or fish) and added to the vegetables or a cup of bouillon. (If someone wants to buy you a gift, ask for a very small steamer pot. You'll use it every day!) Buy a box of unprocessed bran at the supermarket or the health food store, and add bran to your soups, stews, tuna fish salad, and morning cereal. Keep a bowl of fresh fruit on the table for snacking. Be sure to add half a banana or an apple and raisins to your cereal in the morning.

If this regimen doesn't take care of the problem and more help is needed, several natural, non–habit forming stool softeners are available. Docusate (Colace) capsules are recommended and can be purchased without prescription. Exercise is also a very important aid. People with Parkinson's need to exercise every day for other reasons, too.

If your Sinemet is causing side effects such as bloating, cramping, and gassiness, you will want to avoid baked beans, cabbage, broccoli, cauliflower, brussels sprouts, beer, and carbonated beverages.

Many people with Parkinson's suffer from depression caused by chemical changes in the brain, and they lose their interest in eating. If your present medication does not relieve the depression, you may want to ask your doctor to prescribe an additional medication to control depression, so that you can go back to eating well and enjoying life.

An unusual problem that is easy to correct is associated with hot, spicy foods. Some people with Parkinson's report that they experience discomfort, even violent dyskinesias (wild movements of parts of their bodies), after a highly spiced meal. They feel much better when they eat bland or mildly seasoned foods.

Some people with Parkinson's are overweight (although there are far fewer overweight than underweight ones). Perhaps some are overweight because they don't exercise and keep busy and active. A vicious cycle can set in: because they are overweight, moving about becomes much more difficult, and they become even more inactive. But lack of activity isn't always to blame. Although I had always been slim, I began gaining weight steadily a few years ago until I was thirty pounds heavier. I disliked being overweight, but neither dieting nor exercising took any weight off. Finally, I had tests done that showed that my thyroid gland was underactive. With thyroid medication, I've finally been shedding the pounds. If you are overweight and have ruled out a low-thyroid problem, ask your doctor to put you on a well-balanced diet, and start an exercise regimen. Or perhaps you may want to ask your doctor to start you on the Parkinson's "protein redistribution diet," sometimes called the "low-protein diet."

The protein redistribution diet isn't for everyone. If you are seriously underweight, it isn't for you. If you are recuperating from surgery or any type of wound, you are not a candidate, either. And if you have diabetes, you can't even think of trying this diet! But if you are normal in weight or overweight, healthy in all respects except for your Parkinson's, and Sinemet (or another form of levodopa) is part of your drug regimen, you may want to consider the protein redistribution diet. Be sure to consult your doctor, and be sure that he or she knows what you are doing. Your doctor may have to modify your medication very soon after you begin the diet. Your Sinemet may have a much stronger effect, and you may need less of it or you will develop symptoms of overmedication.

What is the story of the protein redistribution diet? In the past, an increasing number of people with Parkinson's reported that they felt better and more energetic during the day if they ate very little protein for breakfast and lunch. These patients ate their whole day's protein at dinner, and because they slept at night, they did not need to worry about a lack of energy after dinner. Researchers looked into these claims and learned that there was a basis for them. They learned that protein competes with the levodopa in Sinemet. The amino acids that make up protein interfere with levodopa's ability to pass from the intestine into the bloodstream; these amino acids also interfere with the ability of levodopa to pass from the bloodstream into the brain. The researchers devised a diet that redistributes the protein that is eaten during the day.

In the protein redistribution diet, only about 7 grams of protein can be consumed during the day until just before the evening meal. During this time period, patients eat foods that contain only trace amounts of protein, including rice cereal; fresh and dried fruits; salad vegetables; cornstarch; jams and jellies; honey, oils, and fats; herbs and spices; vinegar; liquid or powdered non-dairy creamer; crackers made of potato starch or rice starch (but no flour); coffee, tea, lemonade, fruit juices, sodas, and alcoholic beverages (except beer); hard candies, sugar, and condiments. If dieters have a low cholesterol level, they may add an egg yolk or two to the list, because there is no protein in the yolk. (The egg whites, which are pure protein, can be saved for the evening meal.) Not one of these foods provides more than a few grams of protein.

During the day, the diet also permits two selections containing a bit more protein. These selections are from the foods made of grains: breads, crackers, cereals, pastas, popcorn, and rice; and from all the vegetables *except legumes and nuts*. Legumes, which include peas, lentils, soybeans, and dry beans (such as baked beans, kidney beans, and chickpeas), cannot be eaten during the day because they contain most of the amino acid building blocks of protein. Together, the two selections should contain no more than 4 or 5 grams of protein.

The 7 grams of permitted daytime protein enable the dieter to eat a serving of cereal with breakfast, such as a cup of corn flakes or puffed wheat or three-quarters of a cup of bran flakes or rice squares, containing about 2 grams of protein. (Cereal boxes can be checked; they usually show grams of protein per 1-ounce portion of cereal.) Cereal can be eaten with nondairy liquid creamer or apple juice, but not with milk. The daytime protein allowance also permits the dieter to take three-quarters of a cup of cooked vegetables or white rice with lunch (containing about 3 grams of protein). Of course, the dieter may not eat any meat, fish, egg white, milk, cheese, or other milk products for breakfast or lunch.

With such a list of restrictions, what can the dieter eat for breakfast? Actually, breakfast is fairly easy. A glass of fruit juice, an orange, or half a grapefruit can be followed by a portion of cereal (described earlier) in nondairy liquid creamer or apple juice and served with raisins, half a banana, or other fruit, and a cup of coffee or tea. For variety, half of an English muffin with butter and jam or a cup of popped corn (prepared with oil, butter, or margarine) could be substituted for the cereal. Other substitutes for cereal might include a slice of buttered toast or matzo, a small plain muffin with jelly, or a small doughnut. (To aid those of you who are not familiar with the U.S. system of measurement, here are the metric equivalents of American measurements used in the recipes in this chapter: 1 cup [8 fluid ounces] is approximately one-fourth of a liter; 1 fluid ounce is approximately 30 milliliters; 1 solid ounce is approximately 30 grams; 1 teaspoon is approximately 5 milliliters; 1 tablespoon is approximately 15 milliliters. Note that the American measuring cup is larger than an English teacup, and the teaspoon is much larger than the English spoon used for tea. American recipes use volume, rather than weight, for measuring ingredients; thus, a cup of sliced vegetables is the amount that fills the space occupied by one-fourth of a liter. Following the recipes should now require you to do only a few simple conversions.)

Before long, it is time for lunch. The list seems even more restrictive. What can you eat for lunch? You must use a little imagination. A cup of bouillon with a few crackers made of potato starch or rice starch could be followed by a garden salad with dressing, a cup of cooked vegetables seasoned with herbs and dressed with a pat of butter or a bit of olive oil, a dish of stewed fruit or fresh fruit salad, and a cup of coffee, tea, or soda.

For variety, the cooked vegetables could be served in some of the cooking liquid thickened with cornstarch and flavored with herbs. Or the vegetables could be pureed, flavored with seasonings and bouillon, and served as a soup. Cooked or canned green beans could be blended at low speed into a half cup of tomato juice, flavored with oregano and basil, heated, and served as a tasty, thickened soup. A medium-size boiled or baked potato served without the skin, about ten medium-size french fries, or a baked (or steamed) sweet potato may be substituted for the vegetables.

Three-quarters of a cup of cooked brown rice or pasta are other possible substitutes. The vegetables should be different each day to ensure that you obtain all the necessary nutrients.

Another good idea: a big pot of vegetable soup that can be divided into portions and kept in the refrigerator for a number of lunches. Vegetable soup combines the bouillon, vegetable, and starch (crackers) portions of lunch. Here is a recipe for a pot of delicious low-protein vegetable soup, contributed by Professor Judith Green of William Paterson College in New Jersey:

MARGARET GREEN'S VEGETABLE SOUP
(makes about 8 cups)

4 cups bouillon (chicken or beef)
2 cups water
1 stalk of celery, sliced
1 small parsnip, peeled and sliced
3 carrots, peeled and sliced
2 cups coarsely shredded cabbage
1 small onion, diced
2 large cloves of garlic, minced (about 3 tablespoons)
$1/8$ teaspoon ground black pepper
1 cup sliced green beans
2 cups drained canned corn
1 tablespoon salad oil
$1/2$ teaspoon dried oregano
$1/4$ teaspoon dried marjoram
$1/4$ teaspoon dried thyme leaves
$1/2$ teaspoon salt, or salt to taste (if desired)
1 or 2 tablespoons cornstarch (if desired)
$1/2$ teaspoon lemon juice

In a large pot, combine the bouillon, water, celery, parsnip, carrots, cabbage, onion, garlic, and pepper. Bring to a boil and then simmer for half an hour. Next, add the green beans, canned corn, oil, oregano, marjoram, thyme, and salt. Bring to a boil again and simmer for another half hour. (The soup can be thickened by mixing a few tablespoons of cornstarch with a little cold water and stirring the mixture into the soup.) Just before turning off the heat, add the lemon juice and stir well. When dividing portions, mix the soup from the bottom of the pot to distribute the vegetables evenly. The entire pot of soup will contain about 14 grams of protein. If the pot is divided into seven equal portions, each portion will contain about 2 grams of protein.

With a very restricted lunch menu, tasty treats are very important. Fruit desserts can become routine and boring, or they can bring sensational flavor and variety. Fruit salads are refreshing in the summer. Professor Green's favorite is a mixture of sliced fresh mango, chunks of honeydew melon, and blueberries, sprinkled with lemon juice. She also recommends ripe pineapple chunks mixed with seedless orange pieces, sliced bananas, and seedless grapes, served in apricot nectar. Warm desserts are appreciated in the winter. Apples (cored and sliced) can be cooked with a little water, cinnamon, raisins, brown sugar, and a pat of butter and served with a dash of sweet wine. Banana chunks can be baked in orange juice, sprinkled with coconut extract (flavoring) and brown sugar, and served with a dash of orange liqueur. Professor Green offers a recipe for pears:

Sliced Poached Pears
(makes about 5 portions)

3 cups apple juice or cider
2 sticks cinnamon
5 cloves
5 green cardamom seeds
5 firm, ripe Bartlett pears
2 teaspoons lemon juice

Combine the apple juice, cinnamon, cloves, and cardamom seeds in a 10-inch skillet. Bring to a boil, cover, and simmer for about 10 minutes. While the juice is simmering, wash and peel the pears, cut them in half, and core them. Arrange the pear halves (cut side up) in the liquid, spooning some of the fluid over the tops. Cover and simmer for 15 minutes. Add the lemon juice and simmer for another minute or two. Transfer the pears to a serving dish or a storage bowl. Pour the poaching liquid over the pears and let them steep until serving time. Discard the cloves, seeds, and sticks.

One must look for them, but special low-protein breads and low-protein noodles are available for people with special needs. (They are made with starch instead of flour.) Your local dietitian or pharmacist may know where they are sold.

Snacks can be eaten during the day. A snack may consist of fresh or stewed fruit, celery sticks or other salad vegetables, crackers made of rice starch spread with a little jam, hard candies, mints, coffee, tea, or soda. (Diet soda is not used because most diet sodas contain aspartame [Equal sweetener], a protein, rather than a carbohydrate. There is some evidence that aspartame interferes with the medication.)

At last, the dieter looks forward to dinner. Almost all of the day's requirements for protein are eaten at the evening meal. As we learned before, it is especially important for people with Parkinson's to consume an adequate amount of protein. They need to maintain their weight, and protein provides far more calories than carbohydrates do. Also, they need the amino acids that make up the protein, because the amino acids perform many important functions. For example, the amino acid tryptophan raises the level of serotonin in the brain. Serotonin, another chemical messenger of the brain, is thought to be low in people who have Parkinson's. It promotes normal sleep and lowers sensitivity to pain. Another amino acid in protein, tyrosine, increases the levels of dopamine and other brain chemicals that combat parkinsonism and depression. A high-protein meal helps raise the level of tyrosine in the brain.

But what is an adequate amount of protein? The minimum daily requirement for the general population is one-half a gram of protein for every kilogram of a person's body weight.

How do you calculate that? Divide your weight in pounds by 2.2 to find your weight in kilograms. For example, if you are a man who weighs 158 pounds, divide 158 by 2.2; you weigh approximately 72 kilograms. For every kilogram, you need to consume a half-gram of protein: 72 divided by 2 equals 36 grams of protein. If you are a woman who weighs 130 pounds, your weight in kilograms is 130 divided by 2.2, or approximately 60 kilograms; you would need at least 30 grams of protein daily. But the person with Parkinson's needs *more* protein than this minimum daily requirement and must plan his or her dinner and bedtime snack accordingly.

Cooked meats, poultry, fish, and most shellfish, as well as canned salmon and tuna, contain approximately 7 grams of protein *per ounce*. Thus the 158-pound man meets his 36-gram minimum requirement with a portion of meat or fish that weighs a bit more than 5 ounces (cooked weight, not counting the bones). The 130-pound woman needs a portion of approximately $4^{1}/_{2}$ ounces. Milk contains about 8 grams per cup; a large egg white contains about 7 grams; a half-cup of yogurt contains about 8 grams.

People with Parkinson's must not limit themselves to the minimum requirement. At the evening meal they can have as much protein as they wish. In addition to their meat or fish, they can mix leftover hard-boiled egg whites into their salads or vegetables. They can take a portion of cheese with their fish or melt it over their vegetables. They can indulge in a side dish of chickpeas, baked beans, or peas.

What should a typical dinner contain? Perhaps a broiled steak or a large hamburger, served with peas or baked beans and another vegetable, followed by a large glass of skim milk and a slice of cake. Or a helping of roast chicken or turkey, served over brown rice flavored with chopped peanuts or walnuts; accompanied by a salad or a vegetable; and followed by chocolate pudding and a large glass of skim milk. Or broiled fish covered by slivered almonds, served with a cheese-covered baked potato; accompanied by a three-bean salad or a garden salad generously garnished with chickpeas; followed by ice cream or yogurt and a large glass of skim milk. The possibilities are endless. One must only be sure to get enough protein and calcium.

Remember that the protein in meats, poultry, fish, egg whites, and milk products is a much more complete protein than that in legumes, grains, and vegetables. Still, people with Parkinson's need the fiber contained in legumes, grains, and vegetables. They can plan to include legumes and grains along with an animal source of protein. Note that if legumes and whole grains are taken together, they will provide some complete protein: the amino acids not supplied by the legumes are supplied by the grains.

Because almost all dietary calcium comes from milk, cheese, and other high-protein foods, the dieter must be sure to get them at the evening meal and the bedtime snack. A glass of skim milk at dinner and another at bedtime are required. Unfortunately, some people have milk allergies and others have trouble digesting cow's milk. Soy-milk substitutes can be used by people who cannot tolerate cow's milk; in addition, soy tofu and perhaps goat's milk or Lactaid are possibilities. Legumes (such as split peas), the bones in canned salmon, and broccoli are other (lesser) sources of calcium. A calcium supplement (preferably one that also contains magnesium) may be needed.

At the end of the dieter's day comes the bedtime snack. Again, there is no restriction on protein. The snack can consist of an optional sandwich of meat, fish, or poultry; cake, ice milk, ice cream, yogurt, or pudding (made with milk); and a glass of skim milk. A delicious way to take the milk is in a skim-milk shake: 8 or 10 ounces of cold skim milk blended with a half-dozen large strawberries, some crushed ice, and a teaspoon or two of sugar. (A heaping teaspoon of powdered instant decaffeinated coffee and a drop of vanilla can be substituted for the strawberries. Other flavorings and extracts can also be used.)

Many people are concerned about their cholesterol levels. If one's cholesterol level is higher than it should be, the protein redistribution diet can be modified. Instead of butter or margarine, monounsaturated oils can be used: olive oil, canola oil (such as Puritan), and peanut oil. (Peanut oil is somewhat more saturated than the other two.) Salad oils can be flavored with a little sesame oil to impart an exquisite flavor. More fish, shellfish, turkey breast, and chicken breast dinners can be eaten, and far fewer beef, pork, ham, and lamb dinners. Egg yolks, liver, and other organ meats can be avoided, as well as chocolate candy, ice cream, hard cheese, and whole milk. A cholesterol-lowering protein redistribution diet can be managed!

For the protein redistributor, menu planning is made much easier when a list of foods and their nutritional analyses is kept handy in the kitchen. Nutrition books, such as *Applied Nutrition and Diet Therapy* by Grace Burtis, contain these lists in their appendices. (See appendix D7, pages 784–787, in the Burtis book.) Lists can be photocopied from books in the library. The alert shopper also notices the nutritional breakdown (per portion of food) on every jar and package of food in the grocery store. Information from the labels of purchased foods can be added to the nutritional analysis list.

If you have read this far, you are probably wondering, "But does the protein redistribution diet really help?" Research has shown that the diet helps some people with Parkinson's very much, some moderately, and others not at all. Many patients with troubling "on-off" fluctuations are helped. Patients who are resistant to levodopa are not helped at all. The recommendation is that with the doctor's knowledge and supervision, the diet be tried for a week or two. Any benefits will begin to be felt in that time. If no benefits are felt by the end of that period, none will develop later, and the diet should be discontinued. If benefits are experienced, then the person can continue the diet and try adding another grain or vegetable product during the day, then judge whether the benefits are maintained. The doctor may have to reduce the medication of the successful dieter.

Two researchers, Dr. David Riley and Dr. Anthony E. Lang, conducted a study of thirty-eight people with Parkinson's on the

Pincus/Barry Low-Protein (protein redistribution) Diet. The results of this study, which were reported in the July 1988 issue of *Neurology*, showed that patients whose Parkinson's had never been responsive to levodopa received no benefit, but that 60 percent of patients who had experienced "on-off" fluctuations with levodopa were helped significantly. The majority of those who were helped significantly experienced a big decrease in the number of "off" hours during the daytime (before dinner). None of these participants reported that they were any worse in the evening than before they had started the diet.

Among the 40 percent of fluctuators who received no significant benefit, some had very mild reductions in daytime fluctuations, and others had no reduction at all.

One man who did not complete the study developed hallucinations and paranoia. One woman, who did complete the study, developed hallucinations and confusion (a symptom of drug overdose), but this problem ended when her bromocriptine (Parlodel) was discontinued and her dose of Sinemet was slightly lowered. Six patients developed dyskinesias (also symptoms of drug overdose) and, as a result, needed dosage reductions: with less protein, more levodopa reached their brains, and less medication was needed.

An interesting variation in the diet occurred after the study was completed. One former participant who wanted greater mobility during the later part of the day, rather than in the morning, decided to concentrate her high-protein meal in the morning and her low-protein meals at lunch and supper. People with Parkinson's who have obligations or social lives in the later part of the day might want to consult their doctors about following her example.

After the study, some participants who had benefited from the diet tried adding an extra portion of fruit, vegetables, or food made of flour during the day and found that they maintained their benefits.

The protein redistribution diet isn't for everyone. But a nutritious, delicious diet with plenty of liquids, fiber, and sufficient protein should be the aim of everyone who has Parkinson's. With or without the diet, the dosage of Sinemet should be taken forty-five to sixty minutes before the meal.

A large body of research now suggests that a diet with a ratio of 7 grams of carbohydrate to 1 gram of protein is the most effective formulation for maintaining a proper response to levodopa therapy.

Hearty appetite!

CHAPTER 5

Exercise, the Means to an Active Life

Keep the faculty of effort
alive in you by a little
gratuitous exercise every day.

—*William James*

I have found that the more I sit, the more I want to sit. The more I walk, the more I want to walk. And the more I exercise, the more I want to exercise.

Unfortunately, soon after they are diagnosed, many people with Parkinson's begin a sedentary life, sitting in a chair at home. They do this because they think they have to be inactive or because they are depressed. Here are the facts: Parkinson's disease does not destroy muscles; immobility and lack of use do! For people with Parkinson's, exercise is the key to remaining active. Exercise enhances our medication and makes it more effective. Exercise keeps us strong; it keeps our muscles from atrophying. Exercise keeps us flexible.

At the time I was diagnosed with Parkinson's, I was exercising regularly. For some time, I had attended a local exercise class led by a friend on whom the benefits of a regular exercise class were very obvious. In addition to taking the exercise class, I had been riding a stationary bicycle, walking, and swimming. I never got to the point where I was mistaken for my friend, but I was in shape.

My philosophy is that my body is the only one I have, so I must take the best possible care of it. After the diagnosis, I continued the exercise class for two years or more, but exercising that way became more and more difficult for me. I began to look for alternatives. Having retired from teaching, I was free during the day, so I signed up at an exercise salon and used the standard exercise equipment. I also joined the salon's twenty-minute exercise group and did what I could. Then, the salon went out of business. A few years ago, my daughter, Susan, saw an invitation for a free session at a passive exercise salon, where specially equipped tables do most of the work of exercising various parts of the body. Off we went, both envisioning slimmer, trimmer bodies to slither into our new bathing suits. We had a very enjoyable one-hour session, spending ten minutes on each of the six passive-exercise tables. We both joined the salon and eventually lost some inches, if not weight.

I still participate in this program because it fits my needs so perfectly. I try to attend three times a week. As anyone with Parkinson's knows, exercising can be difficult even when the medication is hard at work. When the medication is not working effectively, there are times when I can barely lift my arm. But with the passive exercise tables, I can go any time of the day and feel better when I leave. Even if I'm very tired, I look forward to my time there, as my body relaxes and gets exercised with little effort on my part. These sessions have been very helpful in improving my physical flexibility. After I use the exercise tables, I get the urge to go for a walk or use my stationary bicycle and rowing machine. Then I again start to envision myself as a knockout! (Salons equipped with similar passive exercise tables can be found in many locations; I hope you can find one near you.)

* * *

There are lapses, of course. If my bike and rowing machine could talk, they would tell you about the times they have stood idle. It doesn't take much to interrupt walking and other routines. But I keep remembering that even the healthiest person would become immobile if all she or he did was sit. So I keep plugging along at my exercise routine. Sometimes I'm very good about it, and I'm proud of myself. Sometimes I'm not, and I promise myself I will do better.

Several years ago, Susan and I attended a six-week introductory series of yoga classes. What I learned there has been a big help. The gentle stretching and relaxation techniques help to relieve the rigidity I feel.

Another form of exercise I really enjoy is dancing to music. The music is psychologically satisfying, and in some way it is very helpful. Even ordinary exercising is aided by music.

Walking is excellent for me because it gets me into the fresh air and lifts my spirits.

Isometric exercises are especially suitable for people with Parkinson's.

Parkinson's affects the small muscles, such as those in the fingertips, the face, and the toes. From the outset, everyone who has Parkinson's should practice using these muscles. Pick up little things, such as coins. Play the piano. Sing. Smile a great deal. Blink your eyes.

Even if you are in a wheelchair, you can exercise to strengthen your muscles. You can buy weights that strap onto your wrists and ankles and, while you are sitting, work at increasing the strength in your muscles. You can do some of the exercises in the sitting or lying-down positions recommended for nonambulatory people with Parkinson's. Start with short periods of exercise and lengthen them gradually. Do them when your medicine is working for you, not during "off" periods, or they will do more harm than good.

Physical therapy and occupational therapy are among the most important aids available to the Parkinson's patient. Often doctors wait too long before referring the patient to physical and occupational therapies. The best time to get this help is while you are still flexible, so you can learn how to stay that way. You can get physical therapy at hospitals, at medical centers, or through the local visiting nurse service (check your telephone book).

A less expensive exercise package—a three-ring notebook containing thirty-eight illustrated exercises and two accompanying audio tapes—is available from the United Parkinson Foundation, 833 West Washington Boulevard, Chicago, IL 60607. The cost is $15 to members; $25 to nonmembers.

Several useful publications are available through the American Parkinson Disease Association at 800-223-APDA. They include *Parkinson's Disease Handbook*; *PD 'N' Me: Coping with Parkinson's Disease*; *Be Active: A Suggested Exercise Program for People with Parkinson's Disease*; *Be Independent: Equipment and Suggestions for Daily Living Activities*; and *Speaking Effectively*, which focuses on speech and swallowing problems. APDA booklets may also be downloaded from the Web at www.apdaparkinson.org.

The Parkinson's Disease Foundation offers a free introductory packet, as well as other materials. Call PDF at 212-923-4700, or write PDF, William Black Medical Research Building, 710 West 168th Street, New York, NY 10032. The foundation provides *The PDF Exercise Program*, a three-ring binder with two cassette tapes, at a cost of $15, or the *Motivating Moves for People with Parkinson's* DVD for $14.95.

Begin helping yourself with moderate range-of-motion and stretching exercises today, during your "on" time, working up from ten-minute sessions to twenty-minute sessions, morning and evening. Nurse Linda Perry, of the Boston University Hospital Parkinson's Day Program, recommends a series of exercises in which you move and stretch your neck, shoulders, elbows, wrists, fingers, hips, knees, ankles, toes, waist, mouth, eyes, and all of the muscles of your face. You want to move each of these joints and muscle areas in many directions. For example, when exercising your neck, move your head from side to side, touching each shoulder with it; move your head forward and down to your chest, then back as far as you can, and rotate your head as far as it will go in each direction.

In exercising your shoulders, move them up and down, curl them in and then back. Now the arms: stretch them out to the sides and move them in small circles; move them in and out from the elbow and up and down from the elbow; stretch one arm up, then the other arm up (the whole arm), then both arms up over your head; touch the backs of your hands over your head, exhaling as your arms come down. Make a fist and move your wrists up, down, and around. Stretch your fingers, make a tight fist, then stretch them again. Move your fingers. Massage your hands and fingers. (Even people in wheelchairs can do some of these exercises.)

Exercise your facial muscles: make "funny faces," frown, stick out your tongue, move it left and right, smile, exaggerate long vowel sounds (A, E, I, O, U), blink, raise your eyebrows, massage your face.

Now the knees and the ankles: hold onto a counter or a firm grab-bar, keep your back straight, bend from the knees, and go up and down. Sit down in a chair, hold the arms of the chair, and push yourself up and down. Kick one leg out several times, then the other. Move your ankles around. Stand, hold onto a counter or a chair back, go up on your toes, then down, several times, then do the same with each foot alternately. Walk in place and swing your arms. If you "freeze," break your freeze by imagining a line in front of you and stepping over that line; or imagine that you are marching, and go! Or rock back and forth several times, and then go!

Just a little bit more. Holding onto the back of a chair, bend forward and then back upright several times. Bend to the sides; rotate your upper body. If you have a tendency to retropulse (that is, to step backward), then always keep one foot *back* when standing in place; this will provide a better base of support. Practice getting down to the floor once a day and getting up again. Always walk with your legs about eight inches apart for a better base of support.

For people with Parkinson's, exercising is a must, and it is not that difficult if we exercise only during our "on" time.

This tip is addressed to caregivers. I know that it takes a great deal of patience to stand by and watch someone who has Parkinson's trying to complete a job, whether the job is dressing, folding clothes, or feeding the dog. It may seem that the easiest thing for you and the patient (and the dog!) is to complete the task yourself. It is also the worst thing you can do, because it deprives the person of the movement he or she needs to maintain flexibility. Blaine and I have worked it out so that usually he lets me struggle away. If after several attempts, I can't hook the necklace, fasten the button, or whatever, I ask Blaine for help. There are also times when Blaine sees that I am unusually tired, and he asks if he can help. Encourage people with Parkinson's to be very patient with themselves, to give themselves plenty of time, and to keep on trying. If necessary, leave the room. In addition to the exercise they get in doing things for themselves, there is also value in the feeling of independence they maintain. A sense of independence is very important in building a positive attitude toward life with Parkinson's. And attitude, as we shall discuss in the next chapter, is the key to living well with Parkinson's disease.

CHAPTER 6

Attitude Makes All the Difference

Be not afraid of life.
Believe that life is worth living,
and your belief will help create the fact.

—*William James*

On my desk at school, I used to keep a little clipping that said that when you awaken in the morning, you have two choices: you can be happy or you can be sad, and any fool knows that it is better to be happy!

For people with Parkinson's, attitude is as important as nutrition and exercise. It affects our symptoms. It determines whether our day will be productive and happy or unproductive and depressing. It affects the lives of those around us.

I've learned that I can affect my state of health through my state of mind. For example, many times I've found myself feeling weak and unable, until some pick-me-up comes along and propels me. Surprised, I ask, "How did this happen?" For instance, I may be having an unusually hard time in the morning. I scuffle along and feel incredibly weak and helpless, looking at the housework to be done. I flop back onto the couch. Then the telephone rings, and one of my friends asks me to join her on an outing—a movie, an exhibit, a meeting, a shopping mall, a friend's home, or just a drive. The prospect somehow gets my body moving. I go, and we have a great time!

Once I'm involved in something that is interesting, challenging, or just fun, I observe that I can go much longer without medication and still feel good. (When I become aware that I'm two hours late in taking my pill, my body quickly enters the "off" time.) Medical experts would probably say that the activity acts as an antidepressant, and antidepressants are medications used to treat Parkinson's. I don't fully understand it, but I know that I feel better and like myself more when I have a positive attitude. It's almost as if I get a reward for being happy.

Of course, my state of mind affects my family and friends—and everyone around me. How many times have I heard Blaine say that he didn't know what he would do if I had a poor attitude about Parkinson's. A good attitude doesn't come from wishful thinking alone: we have to work at it.

Of course, we all have bad spells, but learning how to deal with them is the most important thing. For example, after I have done a certain amount of housework and feel wound down and achy all over, I know it is time to sit down and relax with a magazine or a cup of decaffeinated coffee. Or switch to a pokey task that can be done while I'm sitting or lying down. At times I feel depressed. When I'm depressed, I try to spend an hour visiting someone whose company I enjoy. Or I turn on some music and dance (a good pick-me-up) or just listen to it. Sometimes I go outdoors in the fresh air. Or I write a letter or a diary entry. (Writing provides a release of pent-up feelings and helps sort out needs and priorities.)

When I start to say that I can't do something, I try to catch myself and say, "But I *can* do this and this and this." Instead of saying, "I used to do ——," I concentrate on saying, "I'm busy doing ——." I admit that sometimes when I see perky women walking gracefully in three-inch heels, I want to yell, "I used to walk that way before I had Parkinson's!" But the feeling passes, and I swing my arms, step a little livelier, and say, "Thank God for what I can do!" I remember that I am responsible for the quality of my life, for drawing happiness from each day. No one can do it for me, although others can help.

I've noticed that even patients who are confined to wheelchairs can have positive attitudes. An eighty-six-year-old lady came to our support group meetings faithfully for five years, and the last two of those years she was in a wheelchair. Her daughter continued to bring her because she enjoyed the meetings so much. She had a contagious positive attitude. She always said such nice things about her daughter and other caregivers, and they always said such nice things about her. Although she has passed away, her positive influence remains.

Dr. Mark Flapan, a psychologist in New York City, has written with great insight about the role that attitude plays in Parkinson's disease. His article, "Living with Parkinson's: What You Can Do for Yourself," in the Autumn 1989 issue of the *PDF Newsletter*, speaks to each one of us:

Your Mental Outlook Makes a Difference

Even if you or your doctor can't do any more for your disease than you are doing, you can still do more for your life. You can always learn to live better with Parkinson's since how you live with your illness comes from your mental outlook—and your mental outlook is something you *can* do something about.

What's most important in your mental outlook is how you view and judge yourself as a person with Parkinson's. As it happens, how you view and judge yourself can undermine your life as much as your illness can—maybe even more.

Do you blame yourself? You undermine your life if you blame yourself for having Parkinson's. Possibly you believe you got Parkinson's because you didn't take proper care of yourself over the years, or you did something harmful to your body. If that's the case, you know something the doctors don't know, since medical research has yet to find the cause of Parkinson's.

Maybe you believe Parkinson's is God's punishment for bad behavior—although you don't know what you did that was bad enough for you to deserve this. If bad behavior did, indeed, cause Parkinson's, everybody would have it.

I realize that religions have taught that disease is punishment for sinful behavior. If you're troubled by this thought, I suggest you talk to a pastoral counselor of your religion or read Rabbi Kushner's book *When Bad Things Happen to Good People*.

Do you think you're a burden? You undermine your life if you feel guilty because you think you are a burden on your family. Even though Parkinson's has affected your family, it isn't as though you're deliberately doing something by being sick. When it comes to an illness, there is a big difference between *doing* something and *being* something.

Furthermore, it's only by chance that Parkinson's is in your body rather than in the body of some other family member. After all, it could have been your marital partner who got the disease instead of you. But no matter which member in a family happens to get a chronic illness, the whole family is affected, and each family member has to cope with the illness in some way.

Just as you didn't do anything to get Parkinson's, you can't do anything to make it go away. Therefore, you're not responsible for the physical effects of your illness on your family. But you *are* responsible for the effects of your mental outlook on your family, because this is something you *can* change. More about that later.

Do you devalue yourself? You undermine your life if you devalue yourself as a person because you have Parkinson's—if you view Parkinson's as a weakness, a stigma, something to be ashamed of, rather than as a biological happening. Parkinson's, like aging, is something that happens to you, not something you do.

YOU'RE A PERSON—NOT JUST A BODY

There is no question, your body is not what it used to be. You may not be able to do things you used to do: you may talk, walk, and look different than you used to. You may feel stiff, achy, and sometimes in pain. But who you are as a person is more than how you look, how you feel, or what you can do physically.

You're certainly aware of this distinction when you think of how you want others to relate to you. You don't want others to simply react to your changing physical characteristics; you want them to relate to you as a person with an inner life of thoughts and feelings.

You want others to relate to you as someone with hopes and fears, with longings and frustrations. You want others to relate to you as someone whose feelings are hurt when neglected, and whose heart is warmed when shown concern and consideration. You want others to relate to you as a *person* struggling to cope with a disease—not as a *body* that is diseased.

You resent friends and family members who don't relate to you in this way. You resent a doctor who treats you like a "case" rather than a person. You resent a doctor who observes your gait and posture but doesn't see *you*.

But sometimes you, too, forget you're a person and not just an afflicted body. You berate yourself for not having enough energy to do all that has to be done or for being unable to do all the many things you used to do. You get frustrated with yourself when you can't get out a word that's on the tip of your tongue. You get impatient with your slowness. You may even hate yourself because you have Parkinson's.

When you demean yourself in these ways, you're not appreciating yourself as a person—a person trying to cope with a frightening and unpredictable disease. And you're also giving Parkinson's the last word in your life. But Parkinson's doesn't have to have the last word, because the last word comes out of your mental outlook and this is something in your power to control.

If you find it difficult to change your frame of mind through your own thinking, or by talking to understanding family members and friends, or by reading helpful books about living with a chronic illness, you may find psychological counseling to be of help.

You Need Something to Live For

To live as fully as possible with Parkinson's, you have to do more than overcome the thoughts and feelings by which you undermine yourself as a person. You need a purpose that gives life meaning. (The focus in this section on the importance of a meaningful life purpose comes from the writings of Victor E. Frankl of Vienna, founder of Logotherapy.)

A meaningful purpose enhances the will to live, and there is reason to believe that the will to live prolongs life itself. Besides that, a meaningful life purpose counteracts feelings of depression and despair which frequently [accompany] Parkinson's.

You Need to Find Your Own Meaning!

Experiences: Where you find your meaning depends in large part on your past life experiences. Maybe the sights, smells, and sounds of nature made your life worth living. Although you may no longer have the energy or mobility to immerse yourself in nature as you did before, the quality of your experiences, if not dampened by your mental outlook, can be as enjoyable as ever.

Maybe the beauty of music, art, or literature gave zest to your life. Here, as with the experiences of nature, it's not the physical effects of your disease that are likely to limit your enjoyment, but rather your emotional reactions to your illness.

Accomplishments: You may have depended on some activity or accomplishment to make life worthwhile, and Parkinson's may have limited or made these activities impossible. You may have taken pride in what you could do with your hands, and now because your hands tremble you can't do those things anymore. Under these circumstances, you may have to develop new interests from which to derive a sense of accomplishment again.

And if you no longer have the stamina to do all you did before, you may have to set goals that take your energy into account. If you can't do things as well as you did in the past, you may have to reevaluate your standards of perfection. But remember, you weren't perfect before Parkinson's, and even then you didn't get as much done as you thought you should.

But as long as accomplishment is important to you, it's better to continue doing what you can do—at whatever level—than give up entirely on what you did before because you can't meet your old standards.

Relationships: Your life purpose may have come from relationships with people. Maybe there is someone in your life to whom you have special meaning, someone whose life would be diminished if it weren't for you. If this is the case, you have a unique life purpose in relation to that person that no one but you can fulfill.

But you may not feel you have as much to give as you did before. In fact, you may not be able to do as much physically for and with others as you used to. But what you give physically is not nearly as important as what you give emotionally from your heart.

You Can Develop as a Person

If there is any good at all that can come from Parkinson's, it's the potential for becoming a more understanding, more concerned, more caring and compassionate human being.

Since you've been living with Parkinson's, you know what anguish is like. You know what it's like to feel your body changing before your eyes. You know what it's like to feel alone with physical sensations that no one you know has ever felt. You know what it's like to be dependent on others. You know what it's like to live with an uncertain future.

All these experiences, as distressful as they are, can increase your ability to relate to others on a deeper and more meaningful level. What's more, how you learn to live with the limitations and fears of Parkinson's can serve as a model for those aware of your struggle. After all, everyone you know will sooner or later have his own chronic illness to face. (This is so because the miracles of modern medicine cure people of acute illnesses so they live long enough to develop some incurable chronic disease.) How you face your illness may help them face theirs.

Any life purpose that is meaningful to you can strengthen your will to live and enhance the quality of your life as well. Whether you find your meaning through experiences, accomplishments, relationships, religion, a social cause, or some unique path you discover by yourself, depends on who you are and who you can still become. Yes, I said who you can still become. Because even with Parkinson's, you can continue to develop as a human being—a human being whom you value and respect for confronting the challenge of your illness.

Dr. Flapan's article presents a challenge to each one of us: to value ourselves, to pursue meaningful interests and goals, and to develop as people. Think about all we can still accomplish if we set realistic standards for ourselves. Think about undertaking a hobby, whether it is mushroom hunting, ham radio, or amateur astronomy. Think about helping to better the world: join Amnesty International's letter writers and write to governments on behalf of unfairly imprisoned or tortured individuals. Lend your weight to an environmental group that is trying to curb pollutants and toxic chemicals. Tutor a youngster who needs help with reading, or just offer to let him or her read to you once or twice a week. Set up an international student exchange plan in your local high school. Join a Parkinson's support group to help (and be helped by) other people with Parkinson's and to share activities. The possibilities are endless.

I want to end with an excerpt from a piece titled "Mirror, Mirror on the Wall," by Ellen Levin, the eighteen-year-old granddaughter of someone who has Parkinson's (it was published by Parkinson's Educational Program [PEP-USA] in Newport Beach, California):

> I want you to move closer to the mirror, until all you look at are your eyes. I want all of you with Parkinson's to look at your eyes and realize that your eyes have helped you to see life and happiness, and no matter how your outer body appears to others, you've got an inner body. An inner soul that no affliction could ever cause to tremble, a soul that can store all the happiness you want out of life. And it is a soul, your soul, that won't give in to depression.
>
> Finally, I want each and every one of you to smile, force the smile if you have to, but smile, because you're a human being that has the God-given right to seek and secure happiness.

CHAPTER 7

Doctors and Other Health Professionals

Who shall decide when doctors disagree?

—*Alexander Pope*

This chapter is devoted to the search for effective medical care that can help people with Parkinson's maintain their quality of life. Because there are so many health professionals, choosing the right ones can become an overwhelming task. Where can people who have Parkinson's go for help?

I found my Parkinson's specialist through word of mouth. He was recommended by another patient with whom we had come in contact. Other patients whom one meets at Parkinson's support group meetings, conventions, and camps can be sources of information about doctors.

Family doctors can be asked to recommend a specialist. Some may be able to offer an enthusiastic recommendation; others may not. The neurology department at the nearest large hospital or medical center may be able to make such a recommendation.

Among the best sources of information about Parkinson's specialists are the Information and Referral Centers operated by the

American Parkinson Disease Association (APDA). Each center is staffed by a nurse-coordinator and a physician. The centers do not treat patients, but they provide patient services such as referrals, and they distribute manuals, publications, and newsletters. They also work with area support groups.

There are numerous APDA Information and Referral Centers within the United States, and they are located not only in such large metropolitan areas as New York, Chicago, and Los Angeles, but also in less populated areas such as Great Falls, Montana, and Pawtucket, Rhode Island. Eventually, there will be at least one in each state. If you cannot find an American Parkinson Disease Association Information and Referral Center listed in your telephone book, call the association's headquarters at 800-223-APDA for the location and the number of the center nearest you. You can also write to the APDA at 60 Bay Street, Staten Island, NY 10301. (When you contact your local center, ask not only about doctors but also about the location of the Parkinson's support group nearest you!)

Another source of information about medical care is the United Parkinson Foundation's list of movement disorder specialists. The list is based on patients' personal experiences. Write to United Parkinson Foundation, 833 West Washington Boulevard, Chicago, IL 60607, or call 312-733-1893.

Other national Parkinson's organizations also offer referrals. See appendix A for U.S. organizations and appendix C for Canadian organizations.

Once you are under the care of a doctor, you will want to determine how well he or she meets your needs. If you haven't already done this, you may benefit from listing the qualities you want in your doctor and then evaluating how well the doctor measures up to your expectations.

These are my expectations with regard to both specialists and general practitioners: My doctor

- Will listen to me
- Will treat me as a whole person

- Will not rush me
- Will respect my feelings
- Will explain his or her findings and will answer my questions
- Will educate me about my illness
- Will respect my intelligence and have me take an active role in decision making
- Will be willing to refer me to other doctors if their expertise might help me
- Will write up my visit and send me a copy for my records
- Will be available, or will have an alternate who will be available, after office hours in case of emergency
- Will be a person with whom I can feel comfortable

Your needs may be different from mine. We are all different, and we have different needs, but it is important for each of us to determine what those needs are.

The choice of a general practitioner is important because all patients need a general doctor who knows them and knows the overall state of their health. The general practitioner is likely to be the doctor who discovers the onset of such diseases as Parkinson's in the first place.

For general medicine, I have relied on the PROMIS Clinic (in Hampden, Maine) almost from the time it was established in the early 1960s by Dr. Harold Cross. Dr. Cross stresses preventive medicine, and the PROMIS Clinic has a small, efficient team of health professionals that fulfills my expectations. When I visited Dr. Cross with my concerns about Parkinson's, he listened. He didn't brush my concerns aside but called in another doctor for his opinion. Because Parkinson's is difficult to diagnose in the early stages, he arranged for me to see a neurologist as soon as possible.

Of course, the criteria one uses to evaluate the general practitioner should also be used to evaluate the neurologist or the Parkinson's specialist. In your search for the right doctor, do not be afraid to seek second or third opinions or even to change doctors.

Within medicine, as in any profession, some practitioners are outstanding, dedicated professionals; some are average; and some should not be practicing. The patient needs to take some responsibility as a medical consumer in the search for a competent doctor.

Be sure to question the motives of a doctor who gets irritated if you ask questions or if you want a second opinion. If a doctor is more motivated by his or her own insecurities than he or she is by your need for the best treatment, you may want to find another doctor. Remember, if your illness remains poorly diagnosed or poorly treated, *you* are the one who will suffer, not your doctor.

Be alert for the doctor who needs to feel superior and who does so by keeping the patient "in his place." In one way or another, he or she says, "I am the doctor; you are the patient. Just follow my orders." For example, my sister, who had experienced a number of bladder infections, once told her doctor that she needed to see him because she had another bladder infection. He responded by snapping, "You give me your symptoms. I'm the doctor, and I'll give the diagnosis." Another unfortunate incident was suffered by my father during one of his last stays in the hospital. When Dad tried to tell a young doctor about a serious reaction he had had to one of the medications, the doctor left the room abruptly, saying, "If you want to be the doctor, treat yourself!"

Another horror story involved a person newly diagnosed with Parkinson's whose doctor had just prescribed Sinemet for her for the first time: one pill in the morning and one at night. Wary because she had had many bad reactions to medications in the past, she decided to start with only half a pill at a time to see how she might react. The half pill made her very ill, and so did each succeeding dose. She called her doctor to explain that the medication, even a half pill at a time, made her very ill. He responded, "I told you to take a whole pill. You do as I say; I am the doctor." He failed to tell her that a few people cannot tolerate Sinemet at all and that she might be one of them. Eventually, he did take her off Sinemet, but only after he had established who was the boss. Doctors who react this way do not deserve your confidence.

Make sure you are aware of how seriously your doctor evaluates your symptoms, especially if he or she has known you for many years. Does he or she dismiss your complaints as symptoms of "stress," "nerves," or some other ongoing problem? One man shared his story at a support group meeting. Over the course of ten years, he reported symptoms that his doctor attributed to other ongoing problems. One day, while waiting at an airport, his wife saw a man from behind who was slumped over and shuffling along. She thought, "That man is ill." When he turned around, she was shocked—the man was her husband! A visit to another doctor resulted in a quick diagnosis of Parkinson's. A new perspective had been needed.

Remember, the doctor's approach to your treatment is open to your evaluation. Parkinson's is one of those diseases that can be treated and relieved, even if it can't be cured. Through appropriate medication (sometimes a combination of medications) fine-tuned to the individual, physical therapy, speech therapy, and occasional counseling, symptoms can be controlled and productive life can go on. The effectiveness of the treatment depends very much upon the degree to which the doctor and the patient communicate and work together for the best results. Here is a case that really opened our eyes. In the waiting room of Dr. Feldman's office, Blaine and I met an elderly patient whose walk and speech were close to normal. When he was called into the examining room, his daughter chatted with us. She confided that while he had been in the care of another doctor, her father was confined to a wheelchair, spoke only in a mumble, and was very weak (which is typical for someone in the latter stages of Parkinson's) as recently as only one year earlier! Now, under the care of Dr. Feldman, he was in for a check-up before he drove alone to Florida, where he would spend the winter months! Having evaluated his first doctor, he had changed doctors and treatment and was certainly enjoying the results.

That story is much happier than the one I heard on the telephone recently, when a woman called to discuss her husband's life with Parkinson's. The man sits and sits, often staring into space, unwilling to do anything or go out. At his brief medical appointments, his neurologist tells him he is doing fine and that he should come back in three months. I don't know whether the neurologist is neglecting discussion, advice, and the adjustment of medication to this patient's needs, or whether the patient and his spouse are failing to speak up about the patient's symptoms, problems, and needs. I do know that nothing is happening, except that the patient goes home to his chair, the spouse goes back to the same hopeless feelings, and the neurologist goes to the bank with another fee. In this case, as in so many others like it, one can only advise that another doctor be consulted, preferably a specialist in Parkinson's, and that the patient and the spouse take a more active role in communicating their situation and their needs.

I don't want to imply that everyone who has Parkinson's needs to have a Parkinson's specialist to get adequate treatment. However, I do believe that every person with Parkinson's deserves a doctor who has a special interest in (or excellent experience with) this disease, whether he or she is a specialist, a neurologist, or a general practitioner. Common sense tells me that no matter how competent a family doctor may be, no one doctor has the time to keep up with all the new treatments for the broad range of illnesses that he or she may diagnose. The same is true of neurologists, although their area is much narrower. But even neurologists specialize; a neurologist who specializes in Parkinson's disease does not have to divide his or her time among such a large variety of disorders. The neurologist attends conferences and symposia and participates in testing and research that relate to Parkinson's. He or she is aware of all the latest developments and can help patients take advantage of them.

Once you have found the right doctor, you must take the initiative and talk to him or her. Communication is so important! Your health and well-being depend on it. One thing you must talk to your doctor about is the cost of medications, therapies, and fees, as well as the extent to which you are covered (or not covered) in each of these areas by insurance and Social Security. While today's medications and therapies buy you a life span of twenty years or more (up to a normal life span) rather than the three to ten years of former times, they cost a great deal. It is not unusual for a patient's medications to cost more than a thousand dollars per month. If you feel that you cannot afford the cost of some medications, you must talk to your doctor about the best alternatives. He or she may advise a different course of treatment or may advise you to shop around for a pharmacy or another source that offers the lowest costs. (Pharmacies differ enormously in their prices on any particular item. Talk to your APDA Information and Referral Center or to the United Parkinson Foundation about where to find the best buys.)

You are also responsible for informing your doctor of all your symptoms, no matter how minor. And, after following the prescribed treatment, you are responsible for reporting the results back to him or her. Your input is very important in helping the doctor determine whether your symptoms are being controlled, whether you are being undermedicated or overmedicated, whether you are struggling with depression (which can be treated!), and whether you need physical, occupational, or speech therapy. Don't be afraid to bring a list of the points you want to discuss with your doctor, and take the time to cover them all. Write down his or her answers (or ask your spouse or caregiver to write them down)—or bring a tape recorder—if you think you might not be able to remember them. Keep in mind that you are paying the doctor for his or her services.

Lydia O. Cunningham offers some good suggestions in her article "How to Talk to Your Doctor" (*Woman's Day*, August 4, 1987). Some doctors ask the spouse to wait outside while the patient is in the consultation office. Ms. Cunningham suggests that a good response would be, "I'm really not up to par today, and I would like my spouse to stay. I think he can help me to understand and remember what you say better than if I were alone." Sometimes the doctor seems hurried and cuts you off before you have finished discussing the things you planned to discuss. Cunningham suggests that the way to avoid being cut off is to tell the doctor at the beginning of your visit that you have three (or some other definite number of) symptoms to discuss with him or her. Then, if the doctor tries to cut your visit short, remind him or her that you still have other symptoms to discuss. If the diagnosis or the explanation is in medical jargon that you don't understand, ask the doctor to explain it again in plain English. Suppose you are still concerned about certain symptoms or side effects of medications, and the doctor says there is nothing to worry about. Ask him or her to explain to you exactly *why* there is nothing to worry about. Also, ask your doctor to explain the nature and the purpose of any tests, treatments, or other procedures he or she orders for you.

I can't emphasize enough the importance of finding a doctor who will educate you about Parkinson's, who will tell you where to find more information, and, above all, who will listen carefully to you. Because Parkinson's symptoms, progression, and reactions to medication are so different for every individual, the doctor needs to listen to whatever you report and to observe you, in order to prescribe the medications and the dosages that are best for your individual case and to make suggestions about how you might change your daily habits. It would be helpful if, for several days each month, you kept a record of your symptoms each hour, over several pill cycles. Go over the records of these days with your doctor, letting him or her know the types of symptoms you experience and at what point in the pill cycle you experience them. Distinguish between the symptoms of Parkinson's disease and the symptoms caused by overmedication or intolerance to medication (see the next chapter for a discussion of both types of symptoms). Some medications treat certain symptoms, some treat others. Only when he or she is aware of the pattern of your symptoms will your doctor be able to prescribe the most effective medications and the correct doses.

Your doctor should monitor your progress every three to four months. After a change in drugs or dosage, you should be seen every two to three weeks for fine-tuning, until you have achieved the best balance of medication. If you experience bizarre or disturbing reactions, don't wait for an upcoming appointment; call your doctor right away. I have heard the complaint from many patients: "My doctor treats me with 'How are you? Here's your prescription, and I'll see you in four months.'" It's really not possible to treat Parkinson's that way. If you can't get your doctor to instruct you and listen to you, look for another doctor.

Of course, doctors have complaints about patients, too. Some patients don't report all their symptoms. Some don't inform the doctor of all the other medications they are taking. Some patients deliberately minimize their illnesses and symptoms. A few are so solicitous of their doctors' feelings that they don't report the results when a treatment isn't working. Patients need to be open and honest to get the best results.

Parkinson's patients may find it helpful to read the United Parkinson Foundation's pamphlet *The Patient Experience*, which focuses on the things that occur during a neurological examination. Call or write to the United Parkinson Foundation (see appendix A for the address and the telephone number).

Doctors, of course, are not the only components of your Parkinson's medical team. Early in the course of your treatment, and from time to time after that, you should meet with physical and occupational therapists who will teach you important techniques for living with Parkinson's. They will teach you, for example, to walk with your feet well apart—about 8 inches (20 cm) apart—to give you a wider base, which helps prevent falls. They will teach you how to get yourself going when you "freeze" and how to get out of bed without falling. They will help you learn the exercises you need to do in order to maintain your muscles, flexibility, and health.

If you have any problems with speech, a speech therapist should be part of your team, helping you to overcome this impediment. Your ability to communicate is very important to your social well-being. The speech therapist will also teach you to swallow properly so that you don't develop pneumonia that is caused by swallowing food into your lungs.

Finally, a psychologist or a psychiatrist may be part of your team, even if only briefly, to help you (and possibly your spouse and family) accept your Parkinson's and go on with a fulfilling life. A small number of psychologists are specially trained in neuropsychology and are members of the National Academy of Neuropsychology. They are especially able to evaluate, treat, and rehabilitate people with neurological problems; they can guide the planning and the development of educational or vocational rehabilitation programs for people with neurologic impairments. However, don't let the lack of a neuropsychologist in your area discourage you from consulting another psychiatrist or psychologist to help you (and your family) cope with the impact of the changes in your life.

If your doctor has not prescribed these other therapies for you, discuss your needs and ask him or her to suggest the appropriate ones. Or you can contact your local hospital. Also, a visiting nurse service can provide a physical therapist who will work with you in your home. When these services are prescribed by a doctor, they are covered by Medicare and other kinds of medical insurance.

My position is that if I have to put up with Parkinson's for the rest of my life or until a cure is discovered, I want the best treatment that can be found: excellent doctors and therapists and the best medication available. The next chapter is devoted to the medications and other remedies that are available for treating Parkinson's disease. We will take a closer look at Parkinson's as well.

CHAPTER 8

Medications and Therapies

Life is short, the art
    [of medicine] long,
timing is exact, experience
    treacherous,
judgement difficult.

—Hippocrates

When I think of medications that treat the symptoms of Parkinson's disease, I picture in my mind a time line with Sinemet as the focal point. Other medications fall into categories of Before Sinemet or After Sinemet. Most of our knowledge about the treatment of Parkinson's has been gained since the 1970s.

It is important for people to understand the different types of medication that are used to treat Parkinson's disease and the symptoms that each type of medication controls. It is also crucial to know about the side effects. To understand all this, one must first understand more about the disease.

At this time, no one knows exactly what causes Parkinson's disease. Genetic factors may act in combination with environmental factors. Viruses are suspected, and so are chemical pollutants that we eat, drink, and breathe (such as insecticides and carbon monoxide).

A substance known as MPTP, produced in the manufacture of illicit drugs, has been found to cause parkinsonism in humans and laboratory animals. Research with MPTP has led scientists to believe that substances that induce parkinsonism do it by reacting with a chemical in the brain to create other chemicals called *free radicals* that can destroy brain cells.

In any case, something starts destroying the neurons (nerve cells) in a portion of the midbrain called the *substantia nigra* (pigmented substance). These are the neurons that produce a chemical called *dopamine*, a chemical transmitter of messages in the brain, which is sent to another area of the brain called the *striatum*, the area that controls movement, balance, and walking. In the striatum, dopamine counteracts (regulates) another chemical messenger, *acetylcholine*. In the normal person's striatum, dopamine and acetylcholine are perfectly balanced. But with Parkinson's, there is a shortage of dopamine. In the patient's striatum, dopamine and acetylcholine are out of balance—acetylcholine is no longer being regulated.

This imbalance between dopamine and acetylcholine causes the *primary symptoms* of Parkinson's: rigidity of the muscles (stiffness), tremor (shaking) of the hands or sometimes the feet or parts of the face, bradykinesia (slowness of movement), loss of balance and coordination, and loss of "automaticity" (the ability to move automatically without having to think about it). Slowness and difficulties with balance and automaticity are responsible for the problems of falling, festination (short, shuffling steps), sidestepping, retropulsion (walking backward), inability to stop, and inability to "get started." The diagnosis of Parkinson's is usually based on the presence of two or more of these symptoms. Most patients have only some of the symptoms, not all.

To control Parkinson's symptoms, certain drugs can send needed dopamine to the brain; these are the *dopaminergic* medications that contain levodopa (also called L-dopa). Another group of drugs can counteract acetylcholine in the striatum; these are called the *anticholinergic* medications. On the way to the striatum and at the striatum, as well as on cells that project down from the cortex of the brain, there are special *receptors* for dopamine. Medications called *dopamine agonists* can stimulate these receptors to be more efficient. Some dopamine agonists stimulate one type of receptor; others stimulate more than one.

It is believed that in Parkinson's disease, dopamine is also deficient in other parts of the brain. The areas in which these other deficiencies occur may determine which of the *secondary symptoms* a person with Parkinson's may develop. Deficiencies of certain other chemical neurotransmitters may also be responsible for secondary symptoms.

Patients may develop a few (but usually not all) of the secondary symptoms: a stare reminding one of a facial mask, aches and pains, feelings of extreme restlessness, feelings of fatigue, difficulty swallowing (which can cause excess saliva to build up in the mouth, leading to drooling), speech difficulties, shallow breathing, watery eyes, dry eyes, a hunched or bent posture, or prolonged feelings of depression. Still other secondary symptoms may include oily skin, constipation, difficulty voiding the bladder, the feeling of unusual hot and cold sensations (usually in an arm or a leg), sudden excessive sweating, forced closure of the eyelids, dizziness on arising from a bed or a chair, swelling of the feet, and impotence. Various medications can control these symptoms; some can make them worse. (We will take a more detailed look at the medications for Parkinson's later in the chapter.) Diet regimens, speech therapy, and other therapies also help to control the secondary symptoms.

An important secondary symptom is depression, which afflicts about 50 percent of people with Parkinson's. In the past, parkinsonian depression was thought to be merely the psychological consequence of facing life with a chronic disease. This remains true in some cases; however, scientists now believe there is a chemical component—the depression that is so common in Parkinson's may be caused by the same chemical problems in the brain that cause the disease. For years, antidepressant medications have been used both to improve the patient's state of mind and to relieve symptoms. Some scientists are evaluating whether depression in Parkinson's disease may also be caused by a decreased amount of serotonin, another substance in the brain.

There is no typical case of Parkinson's. Each case is different and individual. One person with Parkinson's may develop only a few primary and secondary symptoms, which may be different from those developed by the next person. Individuals also tolerate drugs differently. Each person's Parkinson's must therefore be treated individually, with medications and dosages tailored to his or her own set of symptoms and drug tolerances. Patients who are aware of the symptoms and the medications used to treat them will be more alert to their own symptoms, more apt to report these thoroughly to their doctors, and more apt to get the most appropriate treatment. If a doctor is not a Parkinson's specialist, the patient may even be able to educate the doctor to some extent. Certainly, the patient will be able to explore the options more intelligently with his or her medical team.

Now that you are aware of the symptoms of parkinsonism, you will want to know more about the specific medications that treat them. And you need to know about the side effects of these medications, so that you can tell the difference between the symptoms of your Parkinson's and the symptoms of overmedication and drug intolerance. When you report your symptoms, you will help the doctor and yourself if you distinguish between the symptoms of Parkinson's and the symptoms of overmedication or drug intolerance.

First, when Parkinson's is newly diagnosed and the symptoms are very mild, the doctor may prescribe no medication at all. Until the new drug deprenyl (Eldepryl) became available in the United States in the summer of 1989, it was thought that medication should be delayed until parkinsonian symptoms affected the patient's life too adversely to remain untreated. Deprenyl, also called "selegi-line," was discovered by Joseph Knoll in Hungary in 1964, has been used in Europe for many years, and is marketed in Europe under the trade names Eldepryl and Jumex. (In the United States, it is imported from Hungary and marketed as Eldepryl.) In the November 16, 1989, issue of the *New England Journal of Medicine*, the Parkinson Study Group (Datatop) published its research find-ing that "the use of deprenyl (10 mg per day) delays the onset of disability associated with early, otherwise untreated cases of Par-kinson's disease." The study indicates that deprenyl may slow down the progression of the disease if it is administered early. This research group also found that early treatment with deprenyl permitted patients to delay the need for Sinemet and to continue working at their jobs longer than untreated patients could.

Other research in Europe and the United States shows that deprenyl is also helpful at other stages of the disease. Scientists think that it may slow down the destruction of cells in the sub-stantia nigra, thus slowing down the progression of the disease. With deprenyl, a patient may need less Sinemet. Lower dosages of Sinemet reduce the side effects and permit longer use over the years. For some people with Parkinson's, deprenyl smooths out the "on-off" and "wearing off" phenomena.

What is deprenyl, and how does it work? You remember that a toxic substance such as MPTP can react with a chemical in the brain to start the degeneration of the cells in the substantia nigra. Some researchers believe that deprenyl can block the toxic effect of such substances. Scientists also believe that deprenyl inhibits the action of a substance in the brain called monoamine oxidase-B (MAO-B), which inactivates dopamine. They theorize that depre-nyl stops or slows down the destructive action of chemicals called free radicals that are formed when MAO-B reacts.

The most interesting thing that research seems to indicate about deprenyl is that deprenyl may not merely control symptoms as other Parkinson's medications do, but it may also slow the pro-gression of the disease. It has few side effects, except that it can cause insomnia in some people and can also aggravate an existing stomach ulcer. It can cause symptoms of overmedication in some people, which may mean that less Sinemet is needed. Never use more than your doctor prescribes.

Other substances that are thought to inhibit the destructive action of free radicals are vitamin E and vitamin C. It is thought that these vitamins may slow the progression of Parkinson's disease.

In the early 1990s, even as a five-year Datatop study was testing the value of deprenyl and vitamin E, some doctors were already recommending 400 to 3,200 IU of vitamin E and 1,000 mg of vitamin C. Some people with Parkinson's said that they felt better while taking the supplements.

In June 1993, the *New England Journal of Medicine* reported the findings of the study—that deprenyl was effective, but that vitamin E did not seem to be useful in treating Parkinson's. Four years later, however, the same journal *did* find that either substance could be useful in slowing the effects of Alzheimer's disease.

Do not take large amounts of either of these vitamins without consulting your doctor; if you have blood pressure problems, for example, you may not want to take much extra vitamin E.

Which medications besides deprenyl are used to treat early, mild Parkinson's symptoms? The medication used first may be amantadine (Symmetrel), a drug used to treat flu symptoms. Scientists think that amantadine may help to release dopamine from the cells of the substantia nigra. Side effects in some people include blotches on the legs or swelling of the feet. In a small number of elderly people who have Parkinson's, this drug may cause confusion, delusions, or hallucinations. Another side effect may be dryness of the mouth. If a person has the problem of excess saliva (drooling), then this drug may help to control it. Remember that people with Parkinson's vary widely in their tolerance to different medications. A drug that causes one or more side effects in one person may cause different side effects in another, and no side effects at all in a third.

Other medications to treat early Parkinson's symptoms include the older anticholinergic drugs. You remember that anticholinergic drugs decrease the action of acetylcholine, which is out of balance with the reduced supply of dopamine in the brain. Anticholinergic drugs include trihexyphenidyl (Artane), biperiden (Akineton), procyclidine (Kemadrin), and benztropine (Cogentin). They are especially helpful in controlling tremor. If your tremor is severe, your doctor may add an anticholinergic drug to your medications, because for some people these drugs are more effective than Sinemet is for controlling tremor. They are also useful in controlling early rigidity, but they are not helpful for treating slowness of movement or problems with balance or walking.

The typical side effects of anticholinergic medications are dry mouth, constipation, blurred vision, and difficulties in voiding the bladder. The most disturbing side effects are on the mind: forgetfulness, delusions, or hallucinations. Again, individuals differ in their reactions, and some people may not be affected. If one of the drugs in this group causes difficult side effects, another drug may be tried, and so on. One may work for you with no side effects. A note of caution: When you have your prescription filled at the pharmacy, be sure that the pharmacist has given you the very same medication that the doctor prescribed. There is a practice called "therapeutic substitution," in which the pharmacist is free to substitute a drug of the same general class with a *different* active ingredient for the one that is called for in the prescription. Thus, he or she might substitute Cogentin for Artane, for example. Be sure to check that no such substitution has been made. (Therapeutic substitution is not the same as generic substitution, where the active ingredient is the same.)

Another group of drugs that may also be used in the early stage of Parkinson's includes the antihistamines, such as diphenhydramine (Benadryl) and orphenadrine (Disipal). People with Parkinson's must be careful not to use antihistamines on their own to control allergies, colds, or insomnia: these may upset the balance of the Parkinson's medications and cause bizarre reactions.

Antidepressant drugs are sometimes used in early Parkinson's and beyond. They counteract depression and relieve Parkinson's symptoms as well. Some antidepressants also have sedative qualities that work best for depressed patients who suffer from insomnia. Other antidepressants without sedative qualities are better for depressed people with Parkinson's who don't have insomnia. There are too many of these drugs on the market to name here. Again, these drugs must be coordinated carefully with the rest of the drug regimen. Possible side effects include dizziness on standing and confusion. Changes in heart rhythm may occur in patients with heart disease.

A very important drug that is sometimes started early in Parkinson's is bromocriptine (Parlodel). Bromocriptine is a dopamine agonist, which stimulates the dopamine receptors. It is a limited dopamine agonist because it doesn't stimulate all three types of receptors, but it's very useful in relieving slowness of movement, rigidity, and leg cramping. Some doctors recommend an early drug regimen that consists of an anticholinergic medication to relieve tremor and bromocriptine to relieve the other primary symptoms.

Bromocriptine, taken along with Sinemet, is also useful in the middle and later stages of Parkinson's. But bromocriptine has two serious side effects in some patients: it can cause both low blood pressure and psychosis. Other possible side effects are nausea, involuntary movements, confusion, dizziness, drowsiness, visual disturbances, shortness of breath, and constipation. Because of its possible effect on blood pressure, the first dose should be very small, and increases should be gradual. You can read more about bromocriptine in the manufacturer's own literature. Never increase the dose of this drug on your own, and *never* take it more often than your doctor has prescribed.

Patients who cannot tolerate bromocriptine or who no longer respond well to it may try a newer dopamine agonist, pergolide (Permax). Pergolide stimulates two types of dopamine receptors and is much stronger and longer acting than bromocriptine. It also is especially useful for patients who no longer respond well to Sinemet. Pergolide, too, has possible side effects: involuntary movements (twisting, jerking, and so on) and some cardiovascular problems, as well as the problems listed for bromocriptine. Another dopamine agonist, lisuride, is not available in the United States at the time of this writing.

As most people with Parkinson's know, when their symptoms are no longer controlled by the medications used in the earliest stages of the disease, the next medication is Sinemet. It contains levodopa, the most important drug used in treating Parkinson's disease since 1970. Sinemet is the trade name for a drug that combines levodopa and carbidopa. The levodopa travels to the brain, where it is converted to needed dopamine. The carbidopa stops levodopa from being converted into dopamine in other parts of the body (where dopamine is not only wasted but causes severe nausea and vomiting). Carbidopa is called an *inhibitor* because it inhibits the enzyme that converts levodopa into dopamine. Another inhibitor, benserazide, is combined with levodopa in a less widely used drug, Madopar. With the addition of inhibitors, much more of the levodopa gets to the brain than was the case with earlier levodopa drugs, and smaller amounts of it are sufficient.

Sinemet tablets are available in three strengths: 10/100, 25/100, and 25/250. The top number represents milligrams of carbidopa, and the bottom number represents milligrams of levodopa. My doctor started me on one 10/100 Sinemet per day (one-half tablet twice a day). Then he increased the dose slowly, so that after eight years I was taking three or four 10/100s per day, depending on my needs. Overmedication is a common problem. Remember that you can always discuss your medication with your doctor and seek a second opinion from another doctor if you are concerned that you are being given too many pills, too soon.

Most Parkinson's patients respond to Sinemet. If someone does not respond at all to Sinemet, doctors investigate the possibility that the patient has a *look-alike disease*, rather than Parkinson's. (Look-alike diseases are discussed later in this chapter.) Sinemet, like all Parkinson's medications except deprenyl, controls the symptoms of the disease but not its progression. Sinemet controls the primary symptoms of Parkinson's very well, except that in some people it does not control tremors effectively. If you have a tremor that is interfering with your work or daily life, you need to discuss with your doctor the possibility of your taking an additional medication to control it.

Remember that Sinemet is best taken approximately forty-five to sixty minutes before meals. Observe the amount of time your Sinemet takes to kick in, and schedule that amount of time between taking your pill and eating your meal. Sinemet will work better if it is not competing with your food, and your meal will be more enjoyable when your medication is already working.

Scientists believe that protein (in meat, fish, milk products, eggs, cheese, legumes, wheat products, and nuts) competes with Sinemet and reduces its effect. Doctors now advise people with Parkinson's who take Sinemet and who experience troubling fluctuations to avoid protein during the day (breakfast and lunch), when they need their strength, and to take the whole day's protein requirement at the evening meal. (See chapter 4 on nutrition for suggested meals and menu planning.) The low-protein (or protein redistribution) diet should be undertaken only under the supervision of the doctor, because sometimes people have occasional bizarre reactions to it. The doctor may have to modify the dosage of Sinemet after the start of the low-protein diet. The diet should be designed by a dietitian who is familiar with the needs of the person with Parkinson's and with how to fit nutritional requirements into a very different eating pattern. Patients who are diabetic, seriously underweight, or recovering from surgery or lacerations should not attempt this diet.

Parkinson's patients continue to respond to Sinemet for a varying number of years, some people for many years and others for fewer. One of the biggest problems is that over time, this drug becomes less effective for the patient, so that larger and larger doses are given. As the doses increase, so do the side effects.

One rare side effect of Sinemet is a skin rash or an eruption. A more troubling side effect is called *dyskinesia*. Dyskinesias are large involuntary movements, such as writhing, twisting, jerking, smacking of the lips, or bobbing of the head, all of which are very different from the fine tremors of the disease itself. Another side effect, *dystonia*, is the abnormal posturing of an extremity (a hand or a foot). A very bothersome side effect is the "on-off" effect, in which a person may experience sudden changes in mobility. For example, he may suddenly "freeze" in the middle of a step (which may cause him to fall). Or he may go from immobile to "up and able" in a few minutes. There is also an end-of-dose deterioration or "wearing off." The worst side effects of Sinemet are mental confusion, delusions, and psychosis.

There are several ways to deal with the side effects that result from the long-term use of Sinemet and overmedication. One method that doctors use is to delay prescribing Sinemet for as long as possible. Another method is dividing the total daily dose of Sinemet into smaller, more frequent doses.

For patients who are seriously overmedicated, the *drug holiday* is an option. During the drug holiday, the patient is hospitalized for several weeks, and under close supervision, the Sinemet is gradually withdrawn. Toward the end of the holiday, Sinemet is reintroduced but at a much lower dose. At the lower dose, the side effects are reduced or eliminated, while the Parkinson's symptoms are controlled. Doctors have now learned to better manage the medication so that the person with Parkinson's doesn't become overmedicated. Because of better drug management, there is rarely, if ever, a need for the drug holiday.

For patients who are already long-term users of Sinemet, a dopamine agonist—such as bromocriptine (Parlodel) or pergolide (Permax)—may be added to the drug regimen, which may permit the dose of Sinemet to be lowered and may help in other ways to alleviate the side effects. If one of these drugs does not help, another may be substituted.

One of the newer dopamine agonists is ropinirole (Requip), a medication that is used in treatment before levodopa is prescribed, as well as along with it. By 2001, many neurologists were using dopamine agonists as a first drug for people with early Parkinson's, according to information published in the journal *Neurology*.

Studies have shown that ropinirole can be used as a very effective treatment before doctors resort to prescribing levodopa; also, patients who take ropinirole may require less levodopa. Side effects are similar to those of other dopamine agonists and may include nausea, somnolence, insomnia, dizziness, dyspepsia, and headache.

Pramipexole (Mirapex) is also used in treatment before or along with levodopa. Studies have shown that the patient's "off" time is reduced with the use of pramipexole. Also, patients on pramipexole do not have to take as much levodopa. Side effects, such as somnolence, nausea, constipation, insomnia, and hallucinations, are similar to those of other dopamine agonists.

Yet another dopamine agonist, which needs to be given only once a day, is cabergoline. It is marketed in this country under the name Dostinex.

Despite the possibility of side effects, dopamine agonists have proved to be effective even in early Parkinson's. The drugs last longer in the system than levodopa does and also cause fewer motor complications.

Another category of medications consists of COMT inhibitors. COMT is catechol O-methyltransferase, an enzyme system in the gastrointestinal tract that metabolizes levodopa before it gets to the brain via the bloodstream. Such an inhibitor can be helpful, because it allows more levodopa to be absorbed and more to reach the brain. The result is that a patient may take less levodopa, yet still achieve the desired effect.

One example of a COMT inhibitor is tolcapone (Tasmar), which is rapidly absorbed and has a half-life of about two hours. The use of tolcapone requires biweekly monitoring of liver function by the doctor. Because of certain problems, tolcapone has been greatly restricted by the FDA.

Side effects, in addition to liver problems, are mostly related to increased dopaminergic stimulation. They include dyskinesia, nausea, hallucinations, and hypotension. These side effects can usually be reduced or eliminated by decreasing the amount of levodopa taken.

Entacapone (Comtan) has a half-life of two to three hours and is usually taken with each dose of levodopa. Studies have shown that patients taking entacapone show increased "on" time and decreased "off" time.

The side effects of entacapone are not common and are fairly mild. They are constipation, diarrhea, abdominal pain, and discoloration of urine. Because entacapone increases the absorption of levodopa, dopaminergic toxicity can occur, causing dyskinesia and hallucinations. These side effects can be controlled by adjusting the amount of levodopa the patient takes.

A new drug that came on the market in the fall of 2003 is Stalevo, a tablet that combines carbidopa, levodopa, and entacapone. The medication is designed specifically for Parkinson's patients who have symptoms of "wearing off" that can occur with the long-term use of levodopa.

In addition to drugs, there are other methods of treating Parkinson's disease. In the November 1989 issue of the *American Journal of Psychiatry*, researchers reported successful results of a treatment called electroconvulsive therapy (ECT). Research reports since 1953 indicate that ECT (very different from the older electric shock treatment) may have something to offer older patients who are unable to tolerate increased doses of Sinemet or whose symptoms are unresponsive to higher doses. It may also offer hope to older people with Parkinson's who experience psychotic disturbances as a side effect of their medication and who need to be treated for these disturbances.

While ECT has been used to treat severe depression in Parkinson's disease for some time, the idea of treating nondepressed Parkinson's patients with ECT is much newer. Many doctors consider it experimental and controversial. However, according to Dr. Richard Abrams of the Chicago Medical School (in an editorial in the November 1989 issue of the *American Journal of*

Psychiatry), ECT is "safe, inexpensive, and widely available." He says that in 1985, a group of French researchers reported extremely favorable results in their work with people who have Parkinson's. In 1987, researchers in Scandinavia reported that nondepressed patients had a "significantly longer 'on' phase after the active treatment" with ECT. And in the United States in November 1989, researchers working with depressed patients reported "rapid improvement of motor symptoms" with the use of ECT.

Based on these and other studies, Dr. Abrams theorizes that ECT stimulates dopamine receptors. He suggests that if maintenance doses of ECT were administered every two to four weeks (or another period tailored to the individual) after the initial hospital course of ECT, it would keep patients free of symptoms. (He believes that some patients can maintain their improvement for months before needing a maintenance dose. A patient must be observed over time.) He recommends "brief-pulse, right unilateral ECT," which he says has no undesirable effects on memory: "ECT should have fewer cognitive side effects than levodopa or anticholinergics, both of which are capable of substantially interfering with memory functioning." He suggests that with ECT, the daily dosage of Sinemet would have to be decreased by about half. Dr. Abrams recommends "a therapeutic trial of ECT for every patient with intractable or drug resistant Parkinson's disease, particularly those with the on-off syndrome."

In 1998, researchers from the department of psychiatry at the University of Nebraska reported on their use of electroconvulsive therapy on four patients who had not responded to other treatments. Two of the four people experienced mental or emotional problems during the course of treatment, while two were much improved.

As of 2002, there were more reports of ECT's usefulness in several movement disorders.

Pallidotomy (destroying part of the pallidum surgically) and thalamotomy (destroying part of the thalamus surgically) were quite common in the 1950s because adequate medical therapy didn't exist. The development of levodopa, Sinemet, and other medications greatly reduced the need for pallidotomy and thalamotomy, both of which are neuroablation procedures.

In the late 1980s, when it was found that long-term medications didn't solve the problem for some people with Parkinson's there was increased interest in the development of new techniques for pallidotomy and thalamotomy.

These surgeries are performed using local anesthesia so that the patient can be monitored, thus providing feedback during the operation. A halo-type frame is fixed to the patient's head, and MRI and CT scans are performed to determine the target area. The surgeon drills a small hole into the skull so that an electrode can be implanted. Microstimulation can be used to identify the exact location to produce a lesion with an electrothermal current.

Pallidotomy is used to improve bradykinesia, rigidity, and tremor. Thalamotomy is used to reduce tremor and—to a lesser extent—rigidity.

The television and movie star Michael J. Fox underwent a thalamotomy to reduce tremor on his left side in March 1998. His decision to speak openly about his Parkinson's has contributed tremendously to increased awareness of the disease, in both Congress and the general public. In addition, Fox has formed his own foundation specifically to funnel money to researchers more quickly.

Another surgical procedure, deep brain stimulation, involves placing an electrode in the thalamus, the subthalamus, or the pallidum. The electrode that stimulates these parts of the brain is linked by a wire coming out of the skull (and placed under the skin) to a small, programmable pulse generator beneath the skin of the patient's chest. Unlike neuroablation, this procedure can be done on both sides of the brain to help with movement disorders on either side.

Deep brain stimulation does not require making a permanent lesion in the brain. It can be fine-tuned to meet the patient's needs over the years.

Among the newer therapies for Parkinson's disease are several different types of brain implants. In one type of implant, fragments of the patient's own adrenal gland (the adrenal medulla) are grafted into a part of the brain known as the caudate nucleus. The adrenal medulla is a gland with the ability to produce dopamine. In another type of implant, dopamine-producing tissue from the brain of an aborted fetus is implanted into the caudate nucleus. In a third type of implant, not yet used on humans, animal cells that have been genetically altered to produce dopamine are implanted into the brain of a person with Parkinson's.

At first, medical scientists assumed that the implants acted as mini-pumps, pumping dopamine to the parts of the brain that needed it. Now they believe that successful implants, especially fetal implants, may grow and become integrated into the circuitry of the brain, replacing destroyed tissue.

The first adrenal implants, performed in Sweden in 1982, were unsatisfactory. The first fetal implants were performed in China in 1987, but not much is known about them. In September of 1987, a Mexican team modified the Swedish procedure and reported hopeful results with two fetal implants: one that implanted fetal brain tissue into the brain of a fifty-year-old man and one that implanted fetal adrenal tissue into the brain of a thirty-five-year-old woman. Over time, the results from the fetal implant in the man were said to be better than the results from the adrenal implant in the woman. The Mexican team followed up with implants on 40 more patients and reported marked improvement in 18 of them. Of the remaining 22, they reported that some people showed less than marked improvement, and some showed no improvement at all. They reported that 13 of the 40 maintained their improvement for at least a year. Four patients died.

Scientists elsewhere who tried to duplicate the Mexican results were not able to do so.

In the United States, scientists undertook a multicenter study of brain implants in advanced Parkinson's patients, using fragments of the patients' own adrenal glands. They did not duplicate the Mexican team's hopeful results. There were frequent medical complications: two cerebrovascular accidents, eleven cases of pneumonia, one case of severe depression, and one person who fell into a persistent vegetative state. Brain surgery is very dangerous, of course, and in the case of transplantation of one's own adrenal gland, two complicated operations must be performed simultaneously. One operation removes a section of a rib to allow surgeons to get to the adrenal gland. The second operation, on the brain, allows surgeons to implant the adrenal fragments.

At the 1988 convention of the Parkinson's Support Groups of America (PSGA) in California, I met Richard Hazard, one of the first six U.S. patients to have the adrenal implant, and Don Burns, who underwent the operation later. Both men said that they would do it again. They talked about a sense of well-being that they hadn't experienced in a long time. But Richard Hazard also told us of the pain he endured during his recuperation from this very painful operation. These operations were not a cure.

It is believed that the results from implants that use fetal brain tissue are much better than those that use the patient's own adrenal gland. One example is the fifty-two-year-old man who was the first U.S. patient to receive a fetal brain tissue implant. Although he had had Parkinson's for twenty years, he experienced real improvement in his mobility even a year after the implant. (His surgery was financed entirely with private funds.)

On February 2, 1990, *Science* reported the successful implantation of fetal brain cells (mesencephalic dopamine neurons) into one side of the brain of a forty-nine-year-old man with severe Parkinson's. The results are considered to be the first well-documented and well-verified fetal implant results to be reported. The operation was performed by the scientist Olle Lindvall and a group of other scientists in Sweden, where research with tissues of aborted fetuses is permitted. Before surgery, the man's parkinsonian symptoms were so severe that even with medication, he spent half of his time frozen in four or five "off" states per day. Within three months after surgery, with medication, he was experiencing only one or two brief "off" periods a day and mild symptoms. His rigidity and bradykinesia were significantly reduced. The most marked improvement was on the side of his body opposite the implant. Special brain tests called PET scans (positron emission tomography) showed that the fetal cells survived, grew, and produced dopamine after they were implanted.

Lindvall and the eighty to ninety cell researchers at Lund University in Sweden have continued to make progress in the field.

With the transplantation of fetal brain cells, some patients were able to stop taking medications such as levodopa altogether. Yet not all the patients experienced the same benefits, and some had negative side effects, such as dyskinesias.

And, of course, the use of fetal brain cells remains controversial in many countries, leading scientists to look elsewhere.

According to the BBC, Lindvall told a September 2003 conference of researchers in London that stem cells could be converted into new brain cells to slow physical deterioration.

The hope, he said, was to chemically induce adult cells to change into the type needed for transplant—the dopamine-producing neurons. It would not happen quickly, he added.

More research is needed in this area. Until recently, a U.S. government ban prohibited any federal funding of tissue transplants from intentionally aborted human fetuses. In August 2001, President George W. Bush agreed to allow federal funding for approximately sixty lines of already existing embryonic stem cells.

Just months earlier, scientists at the National Institute of Neurological Disorders and Stroke, a part of the National Institutes of Health, had shown that they could use mouse embryo cells to reduce Parkinson's symptoms in rats. Studies at the University of Minnesota Medical School also showed that adult human stem cells, taken from bone marrow, could be used to make every type of tissue found in the human body.

Not all of North America has been as restrictive about such research. In 1990, the provincial government of Nova Scotia, Canada, reversed its ban on fetal tissue transplants, thus permitting a team from Dalhousie University and Victoria General Hospital to prepare for the clinical trials of fetal tissue implants in four or five Parkinson's patients. Action by the Nova Scotia division of the Parkinson Foundation of Canada, a telephone campaign by local chapters and members, and strong support from the media were largely responsible for the ban's reversal.

Other kinds of research and procedures continue to be investigated. In 1996, Jim Finn of Rhode Island was one of the first dozen people to have fetal pig cells injected into his brain during a procedure at Lahey-Hitchcock Clinic in Burlington, Massachusetts. Two years later, Finn and the successful procedure by Dr. Samuel Elias were featured on the television show *60 Minutes*.

While research on the use of animal tissue continues, the greatest hope may lie in using human sources, whether embryo or adult. Cross-species infection is a concern, of course, with animal tissue. And human sources bring up both ethical and financial questions.

While the federal government moves slowly along this line, private foundations press forward. In March 2002, the Michael J. Fox Foundation for Parkinson's Research announced its bestowal of more than $4 million in grants on two scientific teams from Sweden and seven from the United States, to work specifically in the field of stem cell lines.

The foundation followed up five months later with the MJFF Research Fellowship program, with plans to distribute more than $1 million in two fellowships.

Currently, more than 50,000 Americans are diagnosed with Parkinson's disease each year, contributing to a total of well over 1 million Parkinson's patients across the country.

By the fall of 2002, scientists were preparing to conduct trials for gene therapy, a project that would utilize a gene carried by a virus to help the brain make a chemical called GABA (gamma-aminobutyric acid) that helps to calm tremor. People with Parkinson's don't make enough GABA.

In the spring of 2001, the journal *The Scientist* reported that a DNA advisory committee at the National Institutes of Health had voted unanimously to recommend the protocol, which had proved successful in a study with rats.

Following the gene therapy trials of 2002, the Food and Drug Administration (FDA) gave the go-ahead for human trials based on the work of Dr. Michael G. Kaplitt, of Weill Medical College at Cornell University, and Dr. Matthew J. During, of the University of Auckland.

This advance not only was reported in the journal *Science* but was publicized widely through the print and broadcast media via the Associated Press. Should the trials prove equally successful with people, gene therapy could help countless people with Parkinson's function better for years. Kaplitt and During began a small phase I clinical trial in August 2003, injecting the first Parkinson's patient with billions of copies of a gene into his brain. A year later, the patient continued to do well. A phase II trial is scheduled to start in early 2005.

Just days after the October 2002 announcement about the gene therapy trials, *Archives of Neurology*, a journal of the American Medical Association (AMA), published a report on a sixteen-month study of eighty Parkinson's patients taking either various amounts of the supplement coenzyme Q-10 or a placebo. The double-blind study showed less deterioration in people taking the supplement, especially at the higher dosage of 1,200 mg a day. Members of the Parkinson Study Group recommended a further study using a larger group of patients.

The possibilities for the future are very exciting.

Knowing your disease and the treatments available for it makes you an educated medical consumer. You are an informed patient who can discuss with your doctor the best treatment for you. You can discuss the medications and the dosages used in your stage of Parkinson's and their relative merits for your symptoms. Your doctor should be willing to discuss your drug therapy with you. He or she should be willing to tailor your therapy to your individual symptoms and needs and to supervise you until your medications and dosages are properly balanced.

Discussion with my doctor led to the addition of deprenyl to my regimen and to a lovely vacation as well. In 1986, deprenyl was available in the United States only for patients in the earliest stages of Parkinson's who were involved in experimental programs. I didn't qualify to participate in these programs because I had been on other medications for too long. However, deprenyl had been available in Europe for twelve years, and I wanted to try it. When I discussed my interest in trying deprenyl with my doctor, he gave me the name of a doctor in London, where it was available.

Christmas was drawing near; Blaine and I thought that would be a wonderful time to see London. So I made the appointment to see my newest doctor, and Blaine and I took a week off to fly to England.

Our walk to the doctor's office was very romantic: Harley Street looked like an old English Christmas card. The doctor's office was in the lovely, large parlor room of an old Victorian home. Behind a massive desk sat the doctor, a soft-spoken, gray-haired gentleman whose greatest concern was to make sure that we knew that deprenyl was not a miracle drug. We explained that because of side effects I had already experienced and because I was a relatively young Parkinson's patient, my doctor and I felt that I was a good candidate for this drug. His next concern was the costliness of the drug.

After examining me, he sent me out to his secretary, whose small office was in a space under the stairway. A delightful lady who had obviously worked there for a long time, she, too, was concerned that we be prepared for the cost of the deprenyl. She directed us to the "chemist" (pharmacist), where once more we were warned about the cost. When the prescription was filled, we were surprised (and relieved) to find that the cost was about the same as the Parlodel I had been buying in the United States!

Many people ask me whether I think the deprenyl has really helped. My answer is that since I've been taking it, I've had relatively good years compared to other years that I've had Parkinson's, and I was able to stop taking Parlodel and cut back on Sinemet. I'm glad I had the opportunity to make this decision, and I'm glad we took the step. Besides, we had a delightful week in London!

Knowing the importance of the right treatment, you need to continue educating yourself about the latest developments in the treatment of Parkinson's. Keep up with current findings by reading, attending conferences and conventions, joining a support group, and asking questions. In order to underline the need to educate yourself about your disease, your doctor, and your treatment, I want to share with you the story of Faylene Otis. Faylene is a friend of ours, in her sixties. We take her with us to Boston for her appointment with Dr. Feldman, which is always scheduled the same day as mine. Gradually, we have heard her story, which, I assure you, is not unusual.

When Faylene was a child, she always felt out of balance. As she grew, people often told her to pick up her feet. By 1975, in her early fifties, not only were her feet dragging, but she was always tired. In 1978, she was in an auto accident. During the same year, while attending college courses, she noticed problems with her handwriting, writing shorthand, and shaking hands with people. She fell often, and in August 1978, she fell and crushed her knee. The latter problems were blamed on the auto accident. Later, Faylene was puzzled when she noticed in a family picture that her face wore a frozen-masked expression that made her look "like one of the Flintstones." She knew that she had been very happy at the time.

In 1980, Faylene's local doctor told her that she had Parkinson's disease. He said that she could continue working at her job in the state library with the help of the medication Sinemet. He started her on two 10/100 pills a day and continually increased the dosage so that by the end of six months, she was taking seven Sinemet pills of 25/250 strength—a total of 175 mg of carbidopa and 1,750 mg of levodopa each day. Her body couldn't cope with such a large amount of Sinemet, but no one seemed to realize that. While trying to work at the library, she had to contend with uncontrollable involuntary movements, slurred speech, and the fear that her supervisor would stop by and see her at her worst, which was in the afternoon. She was embarrassed because her condition made her seem drunk—as people with Parkinson's are often thought to be when they lose their balance and stagger.

After six months, when she had become very lightheaded and dizzy and exhibited extreme shaking, her doctor grew concerned and put her in the hospital for observation. But after her stay there, she went home with all of the same problems.

Faylene learned about Dr. Feldman during a trip to Boston with her sister. Discouraged about her condition, she resolved to see him. Dr. Feldman educated her about Parkinson's disease and encouraged her to undergo a drug holiday at the hospital, for she was obviously overmedicated. Faylene agreed and spent three weeks at the Boston Medical Center under close supervision of the Parkinson's team, as the Sinemet was gradually withdrawn. Although she experienced mobility problems during the withdrawal and afterward, her mobility was restored with the help of physical therapy and determination.

When Faylene left the hospital, she was taking one-half of a 25/250 pill four times daily—a total of 50 mg of carbidopa and 200 mg of levodopa—approximately one-ninth of her previous dose. Her speech was no longer slurred, her balance was greatly improved, her tremor was diminished, and she felt much better. She was encouraged as she looked toward the future.

Faylene is the kind of person who doesn't just sit back and wait for something good to happen. If she were, she would probably be an invalid today instead of a traveler planning to visit relatives in Texas. She was not unhappy with her first doctor, but she didn't hesitate to consult another when she realized that the treatment wasn't working for her.

As a Parkinson's patient, you should expect to receive appropriate medication, in dosages adjusted for you, that will result in productive living.

Are you a patient whose diagnosis is Parkinson's, but whose anti-parkinson medication gives you little or no relief from your symptoms? Is Sinemet of no use to you? Unfortunately, there are a number of look-alike diseases with symptoms similar to those of Parkinson's. Diagnosis of these look-alikes may be very difficult, despite new technology such as the PET scan, which can measure dopamine content and dopamine receptor activity in the living brain, and the MRI scan (magnetic resonance imaging), which may help to distinguish between different types of parkinsonism.

One condition of the elderly that may be mistaken for Parkinson's is *benign essential tremor*. This is simply a tremor of the hands and possibly the head but not the legs. Unlike the resting tremor of Parkinson's, benign essential tremor increases when the patient reaches out for something or moves his or her hands. Certain drugs help to control this tremor, but they are different from the drugs that treat the tremor of Parkinson's. Patients with benign essential tremor may wish to contact ITF (International Tremor Foundation), a national foundation devoted to their needs. It was founded in 1988 and has over 42,000 members. You can reach ITF at the address of the United Parkinson Foundation (see appendix A).

Shy-Drager syndrome is a Parkinson's look-alike that starts with dizziness on standing, bladder difficulty (ranging from incontinence to difficulty voiding), and impotence, which are only later followed by the primary symptoms of Parkinson's.

An unusual look-alike is *normal pressure hydrocephalus*, in which fluid cavities in the brain become enlarged. The pressure that is exerted on several brain centers causes difficulty in walking, problems of urinary incontinence, and symptoms of senility. This condition does not respond to medication. (A tube can be placed in the brain to shunt off the excess liquid.)

A disease that is very difficult to diagnose is *striatonigral degeneration*, because it looks so much like Parkinson's. However, in this disease, most of the damage is in the striatum, not in the substantia nigra. Patients do not develop tremor, but they do develop rigidity, slowness of movement, and problems with walking and balance. Their symptoms do not respond to Sinemet or any other form of levodopa.

Arteriosclerotic palsy (pseudobulbar palsy), the result of many small strokes in patients with high blood pressure or diabetes, is another look-alike. Patients may be unaware of these small strokes, but the damage caused to the brain affects balance and walking. Antiparkinson medications do not control the symptoms of this condition.

Progressive supranuclear palsy is a look-alike that causes paralysis of the movements of the eyes, speech problems, rigidity, and symptoms of senility. It does not respond to antiparkinson medications.

Wilson's disease, which causes copper to accumulate in the liver and the brain, appears in patients under forty years of age. (This disease can be controlled effectively if it is diagnosed early enough.)

An unusual look-alike called *olivopontocerebellar degeneration* causes difficulty with balance and walking, and possibly tremor, but no rigidity or slowness of movement. It does not respond to antiparkinson medications.

Dystonia is an inherited, progressive disease (that begins in childhood), in which unusual postures develop in the head, the arms, the legs, and the body. Another form of dystonia that affects only the head and the neck begins in adulthood.

Brain tumors can sometimes be confused with Parkinson's disease. Today, CAT scans or MRI scans are used to rule out the possibility of a brain tumor.

Are patients ever misdiagnosed? Yes, sometimes they are. I have included this information about diseases that are sometimes diagnosed as Parkinson's disease for people who have doubts about their diagnosis or the efficacy of their medication. If you have been diagnosed as having Parkinson's, but your medications, particularly Sinemet, haven't helped your symptoms, you owe it to yourself to get the opinion of another neurologist or a Parkinson's specialist.

In conclusion, I want to mention that because the information for this chapter (except for anecdotal material) comes from medical and scientific literature, you can turn to the list of sources in the appendixes if you wish to know more about any of the topics.

CHAPTER 9

Spouses—
Special and Otherwise

What greater thing
is there
for two human souls
than to feel that they
are joined for life . . .
to strengthen each other
in all sorrow,
to minister
to each other
in all pain,
and to be
with each other
in silent
unspeakable memories. . . .

—George Eliot

Not all caregivers are spouses. In this chapter, however, I want to concentrate on the role of the spouse as caregiver, for the benefit of both those with Parkinson's and their spouses as they adapt to the changes they encounter in their lives. (Of course, some of this chapter is also applicable to the relationship between people with Parkinson's and other caregivers, including adult children.)

The spouse I know best, of course, is my husband, Blaine—who is mostly very special but is sometimes "otherwise" (to keep him human). Let me tell you a little more about him.

When I met Blaine during my college years, we were part of a group that ate together, so we saw each other regularly. At first, I thought that he took life much too seriously to suit my temperament. As time passed, though, I learned more about him. I learned that he came from a long line of hardworking carpenters known for their honesty, patriotism, and helpfulness to others. I saw that he had learned responsibility early, helping at home, cutting timber with his father from the age of twelve, working in a grocery store during high school, and working his way through college. The longer I knew him, the more apparent his many good qualities became and the more things we seemed to have in common. We grew to love each other.

In 1952, we made the lifelong commitment of marriage, and at the same time, we embarked on our careers. After two years in the army, and after graduating from college, Blaine spent several years in school administration. When he decided that he preferred teaching, he taught social studies in the high school and served as the social studies curriculum coordinator. Throughout the years, he did carpentry on the side. When he retired from education, he returned to carpentry full time, forming a partnership—Atwood Builders—with our son, Randy. Recently, he and Randy brought our son-in-law, Keith, into the business as the third partner. It's a real family business!

Blaine is very special, but he's human. I call him "my workaholic." He's never learned when to stop working and just relax. When he's overtired, he gets grouchy. (On vacations, it's good to see him relax the minute we start down the road in our Winnebago.) He wants things to go his way. He worries for the whole family—I've always said that I don't have to worry because he does it for me. He's a bit negative, but he works on becoming more positive. Nevertheless, Blaine's personal strengths stand out.

Our marriage has been solid and good. Blaine is very much his own person, just as I am my own person, which is important. I believe that each partner has to have a strong identity and a good deal of self-esteem to bring to a marriage, in order for the marriage to work.

The "we" has been strong in our marriage. We were in the same profession, most of the time working in the same school building. We took the children camping. We planned and built our home. We decided that I should retire. We decided that he should retire. We decided to buy a Winnebago and do some traveling. We enjoy each other's company, and we appreciate the time we have to ourselves. We both value our good friends and our families.

Soon after I was diagnosed as having Parkinson's disease, Blaine took my hand and said, "You don't have Parkinson's alone. *We* have it, and we will cope with it together." How reassuring those words were! Blaine's message was in character. We knew we were "joined for life," and that together we would face anything that affected either of us. Still, Blaine sensed that I needed to hear him say it. Of course, at that time, Blaine had no way of knowing the extent of the change that "our" Parkinson's would make in his life as well as mine.

Dr. Feldman once mentioned to us that every time he has a patient who is doing really well, he finds that the patient has special support at home. Special support is what I have from Blaine.

Blaine's unostentatious type of support reassures me and tells me that he is sincere. The last thing a person with Parkinson's needs to worry about is her or his spouse's feelings toward her or him. Blaine encouraged me to work on this book. When he finds the dishes still in the sink, he stacks them in the dishwasher. He has done so much laundry that he is beginning to call it "my laundry" (this amuses me because he used to say, "I did *your* laundry for you"). He vacuums the carpets. He makes good salads. When he gets home from work, he's quick to notice how I've survived the day. If he thinks I'm too tired to prepare supper, he suggests that we eat at a nearby restaurant. He is alert to times when I might need a hand but is thoughtful enough to wait for me to give him the okay. His concern is obvious.

Out of concern, Blaine becomes a bit overprotective at times. When I see this happening, I bring it to his attention, and we talk about it. Sometimes the discussion becomes an argument. He feels that I should appreciate his concern. I feel that he has to respect my judgment. For example, he is concerned about my driving the car in bad weather. One bitterly cold day after an early morning exercise session, I decided to go to the library, and I stayed there all morning. Blaine happened to come home very early that day and didn't find me. He waited with increasing anxiety, worrying about how I was coping with the car in the extreme cold. He had no way of contacting me because he didn't know where I had gone. When I finally returned, we discussed the situation. Blaine had been very worried. I wanted him to respect my judgment about when to go out, but I could understand his concern. To allay his fears while maintaining my independence, I promised that in the future I would leave a note or leave word about my destination with our daughter-in-law, Debbie, or our daughter, Susan.

A special spouse plays an important part in helping the person with Parkinson's retain a good self-image. I'm sure that I'm not the only one who feels clumsy at times. When I forget to stand up straight, Blaine sometimes reminds me that I am slumping. He also compliments me when I have dressed nicely or when it is apparent that I have made an extra effort to keep up a good attitude.

Whenever Blaine and I attended conventions of the Parkinson's Support Group of America, meetings of the Capitol Area Parkinson's Support Group in Maine, or our own Greater Bangor Parkinson's Support Group, we were always impressed by the devotion of the spouses of people with Parkinson's. Obviously, the ones who make the effort to attend are most likely to have positive attitudes. But there must be many other devoted spouses who have never been to a support group. Membership in such a group is so important for people with Parkinson's, as well as for their spouses.

Blaine and I have had the opportunity to know and observe many wonderful, caring spouses.

A spouse we have known for several years is the wife of a man who has had Parkinson's for many years; he is also handicapped by blindness. Despite growing difficulties, the wife had kept the husband active and busy for a long time, visiting friends, eating lunches out, and driving to places of interest. Recently, the time came when getting him in and out of the car became very difficult for her, and leaving him alone at home was inadvisable. She found little time for recreation or for herself.

Fortunately, she was not the sort of person to sit at home and play the martyr. She contacted area agencies to find out whether help might be available. First she found an adult day-care center, which he attended for only a short time. Such a center would be ideal for many people with Parkinson's, but it was inappropriate for him because his blindness prevented him from participating in many of the activities. Then she found RSVP (Retired Senior Volunteers Program) and learned that volunteers were available to come and spend some time with her husband, take him for a ride, eat out, or accompany him in whatever he might want to do. This was the program she chose. It gives her time to herself for shopping, visiting, or just relaxing alone. In addition, she takes advantages of offers from family and friends who are pleased to be able to help. One recent morning, for example, a friend took her husband to his lakeside home for the day. We all need to learn how to receive help, as well as how to give it.

It is important to remember that caregivers have needs. Research shows that about one-third of the wives who help their husbands to feel better after heart attacks become so depressed and anxious themselves that they need therapy. (See *Social Support: An Interactional View*, by Barbara Sarason, published by John Wiley & Sons, Inc.) In trying to keep their husbands from getting upset, the wives give in to all of their husbands' demands or hide their own anger, rather than asserting themselves when conflicts arise. I believe that this is likely true of many spouses of people with

Parkinson's. They must recognize their own needs and feelings, as well as those of the patient, and establish a balance. And they must develop a support system of people with whom they can discuss their feelings openly, such as family members, friends, a therapist, or a minister.

Caregivers must also remember that they are not superwomen or supermen. They must be realistic about what they can and can't do. They can't do it all themselves. And they certainly need to allow some time for their own activities. Caregivers will want to read *Mainstay: For the Well Spouse of the Chronically Ill*, by Maggie Strong. Another resource is the Well Spouse Foundation at 30 East 40th Street, PH, New York, NY 10016; phone 212-685-8815; e-mail wellspouse@aol.com. The organization also has its own Web site at www.wellspouse.org.

At the other end of the spectrum are spouses (or other caregivers) who are not constructive in their attitudes and behavior. Their thoughtlessness makes a desirable adjustment to life with Parkinson's extremely difficult or impossible. We have heard people say that their spouses cannot accept their Parkinson's, and we have heard spouses say, defiantly, that they have to go on living as they have always lived. We have seen some spouses build themselves up at the expense of their mates who have Parkinson's. Some are wonderful in public but fail to carry through at home. Some are wonderful at home but are uncomfortable or embarrassed in public. Some spouses take over in social situations, doing all the talking for their mates, as if people with Parkinson's can no longer speak or think for themselves.

These behaviors are disabling to both parties. The person with Parkinson's, left to cope with so many changes with little or no spousal support, feels bereft, rejected, and lost. Even with the support of other relatives and friends, no one can take the place of a spouse. As the person with Parkinson's feels her spouse growing further away, her deepening depression intensifies her symptoms, which causes her spouse to withdraw even further. It's a destructive cycle!

Can anything break this cycle? Psychological counseling is beneficial for both the person with Parkinson's and the spouse—at the outset and from time to time over the years. But with or without counseling, the partners must communicate with each other at home: they must confront problems, discuss feelings, and look for answers. Both partners need to communicate; it is important that neither one gives up in the effort.

Even problems between devoted couples need to be aired and resolved. One couple we know was able to solve a lingering problem by communicating openly. Both partners were retired and generally enjoyed their time together; however, the husband with Parkinson's felt that his wife involved him in more social activities than he could cope with. Through discussion he learned that most of the time, to her he *appears* to be able even when he feels very limited. She learned that even if he *seems* able, he may not actually be able to undertake as many activities as she plans. Together they realized that they could do with fewer planned activities; they could undertake activities when the husband felt up to them.

Problems can be psychologically damaging if they are not understood and resolved. We have heard of caregivers who berate people with Parkinson's for not being able to do for themselves on a given day what they were able to do perfectly well, unassisted, the day before. It is vital for people with Parkinson's to have confidence that their caregivers will listen and understand when they explain that "on-off" periods are characteristic, that there are better and worse days, and that there are even times of the day when the medication works more effectively than at others. It is also vital for the person who has Parkinson's to be able to communicate his or her feelings: "I feel demoralized when you berate me for something I can't control or change. Let's discuss this."

The advent of any chronic disease into a person's life causes extreme worry. At one of our Parkinson's support group meetings, we discussed our worries. The people with Parkinson's all agreed that we worried more as the disease progressed, and the primary worry was centered on the dependency we felt on our spouses or principal caregivers. In this group, where spouses and caregivers are very devoted, one of the main questions was, "What would happen if my spouse/caregiver died first?" Among other people whose caregivers were not as devoted, the additional unspoken worry (whether a basis exists for it or not) was, "What will I do if my caregiver abandons me?" Intense worry affects the symptoms of Parkinson's disease adversely. Sincere reassurance is crucial to the patient's physical and mental well-being.

Although we should not make generalizations (because we are all different), I expect that one of the concerns common to most patients and their spouses is the effect that Parkinson's may have on the marriage. Of course, any change in circumstance will probably have some effect on one's marriage, whether that change is due to a move to a new location, a new member of the family, a new job, a financial windfall or setback, or a chronic illness. Certainly, having to live with a chronic illness puts a strain on any marriage. But if the relationship was strong before the illness, it will withstand the additional stress.

Men and women cope differently with changes in their lives. For example, the prospect of early retirement may be extremely difficult for men who feel responsible for earning the family's living. Many men, especially older men, have been conditioned to feel that they must be strong. The arrival of Parkinson's into their lives may result in feelings of weakness and loss of control. Such feelings can impact on a marriage if they are not confronted, discussed openly, and resolved in some mutually acceptable way.

I believe that in general, one's marriage will be as good or as poor as it was before Parkinson's. Don't expect your spouse to become more loving because you have Parkinson's. He is what he is. She is what she is.

Nevertheless, in any marriage there are opportunities for growth and insight; often a major change in circumstance is just what creates these opportunities. The partners are shaken out of their routine existence and prompted to take a fresh view of their goals, activities, and lives. They reevaluate what is really important to them. They dig a little more deeply within to see what they can contribute and how creative and innovative they can be. Complacency is replaced by new, fresh thinking and constructive action. Sometimes a marriage counselor can be of assistance. But couples embarking on this effort themselves, especially with the help of support groups, can accomplish much. In the process, both partners grow, discovering new potential within themselves and new resources that they never recognized before.

Adopting a positive attitude and keeping communication open are essential to sustaining a good marriage; problems get solved that could otherwise beset the marriage.

For example, many couples facing the spouse's need for retirement and the resultant loss of income have examined their fears together, assessed their finances, opted for a less expensive home and lifestyle, and found that they enjoyed their leisure and many new activities together.

One of the most pressing questions in the minds of people who were newly diagnosed with Parkinson's and their spouses is, "How will Parkinson's disease affect our sexual lives?" Very little has been written on this topic, and very little is mentioned in doctors' offices. The majority of doctors never introduce the subject, and most couples are too reticent to ask about it. Friends joke but don't discuss it seriously (although women are more likely to talk about it with close female friends than men are with male friends). Unfortunately, if you can't talk to your spouse, your chances of talking it over with anyone else are extremely limited. A lack of openness between the partners could lead to second-guessing and hurt feelings: "Am I unattractive to him now?" "Is she afraid of catching it?" "Does he think I don't enjoy sex any more?" "Does she think I'm not physically able to perform sexually?"

From what little is known, here are some basic facts: Parkinson's disease is not transmitted through sexual relations. Of the 1.5 million people with Parkinson's in the United States, only a very few have spouses who have developed Parkinson's. The number is so low that chance, rather than intimacy, is responsible for these few couples. That is, each of the partners would have developed Parkinson's no matter whom he or she married; one did not "catch it" from the other.

It is well known that the decreased mobility caused by Parkinson's can affect sexual function. The more rigidity and immobility there is, the more difficult any physical activity will be. However, when Parkinson's is treated with Sinemet, rigidity decreases and mobility increases; most patients treated with Sinemet enjoy an improvement in their sexual lives. The drug deprenyl also has an enhancing effect. (It is interesting that in addition to slowing the progress of Parkinson's, deprenyl has been shown to slow the general aging process in laboratory animals and to preserve physical functions, including sexual function. In the future, research will show whether deprenyl has any effect on the aging process in humans.)

Some drugs have the opposite effect: Artane and certain antidepressants used to treat Parkinson's can have an adverse effect on potency in men and libido in women.

Most people with Parkinson's are either elderly or in the upper middle years, a time when hormones, desire, and energy normally wane to some degree, with or without Parkinson's disease. Sexual needs do change gradually for everyone. Even though many older people enjoy an active love life, most notice a decrease in the amount of energy they seem to have and an increase in aches and pains. Hard work, emotional stress, and the prospect of retirement all affect sexual performance. It's easy to blame Parkinson's when aging and other factors may be operating.

A satisfactory sexual life is possible with Parkinson's when the disease is treated properly. I believe that in general, the kind of sexual relationship that partners had before Parkinson's will determine the kind of relationship they'll have with it. If they had open communication about their sexual needs before and continue to have open communication, there is no reason for their sexual relationship to change.

One of the very few essays in print that addresses the topic of sexuality and Parkinson's disease contains several sections written by Dr. George W. Paulson, the chairman of Neurology at Ohio State University Medical School, and other sections were written by Joseph L. Howard, the husband of a Parkinson's patient (see *United Parkinson Foundation Newsletter*, 1985, no. 4, part 2). Dr. Paulson's comments are frank and straightforward:

> There is no reason that sexual intercourse is dangerous for patients with Parkinson's disease. . . . Parkinson's disease does lead to stiffness of the back and limbs, and movements which were once reflexive or automatic have to come under conscious control.

About men with Parkinson's, he writes,

> It may be that the female will have to become more active, perhaps assuming an on-top position. It may even be necessary to use alternatives to traditional intercourse, such as oral or manual stimulation. The remarkable fluctuations some patients have can perplex the wife. Sometimes the man is quite adroit and at other times can, at best, be a passive recipient of her attention to their mutual needs.

He also says,

> Certainly, . . . impotence is very common in Parkinson's disease patients. Additions of testosterone or male hormones are not usually helpful. [A urologist can offer information about penile implants and other mechanical aids.] Secondary impotence should also be considered. This implies that after a failure or a limited success, the man develops a psychologic block. Fear of nonperformance, worry about the partner's response, a sense of depression or guilt can, of itself, lead to impotence. The wife . . . [in attempting to spare her husband any further upset] may withdraw or refuse to try. If sexual activity is discontinued for long periods of time, it may be very difficult to resume. . . .

[However], the impotence in Parkinson's disease is generally organic, not psychologic.

In any case, the man with Parkinson's who experiences impotence is advised to see a urologist. About women with Parkinson's, Dr. Paulson says,

> Some women with Parkinson's disease will, of course, lack lubrication to such an extent that clitoral stimulation will be painful. Anticholinergics which produce such drying of the mouth may not dry the vagina so markedly. At times, painful uterine contractions can occur, or there can be a nagging pelvic pain that produces fear and inhibition in both partners.

For women who are not familiar with these products, K-Y Jelly and hormone creams are useful lubricants. Consult a gynecologist about them. After menopause, even women who do not have Parkinson's find that they need commercial lubricants. Dr. Paulson also says,

> There has been no study which suggests inevitable decline of orgasmic ability in women with Parkinson's disease, but since Parkinson's disease does affect the autonomic nervous system, it seems quite possible that orgasm and intercourse will usually become less free as the disease advances.

Dr. Paulson concludes with this reminder:

> Love is more than sex. I have more patients complaining about lack of closeness or lack of verbal communication than about lack of sexual skills or opportunity. Fortunately, however, partners with Parkinson's disease have usually retained their loyal spouses and have a life-time of devotion to sustain one another. . . . Talking, fondling, hugging, touching, and shared sensual experiences of many kinds can continue to enrich a couple, no matter how disappointing the decline in sexual activity may be. "For better or worse" still includes a lot of "better"—you just have to look a little harder for it.

The reader must keep in mind that the article quoted here was written in 1985. More recent medications and therapies may have a favorable effect on all physical functions.

It is important to keep things in perspective. Many people think only of sexual intercourse when the word *sex* is mentioned. Actually, it is a small part of sexuality. A marriage counselor who often spoke to the students in my Marriage and Family class at school used to say that it is easy to have intercourse; developing a meaningful sexual relationship is what takes time, effort, and maturity. Both the person with Parkinson's and the spouse still have the same needs as before, including the need to be desirable to each other; the need for hugs, kisses, and cuddling; the need for intimacy and the loving touch. Express yourself openly to your spouse—and be a good listener. Be willing to explore, both verbally and physically. Only then can you make sure that you are not cheating yourself out of a satisfying sexual relationship.

Over the eighteen years that I've had Parkinson's, we've seen many changes. Therefore, my husband has made many adjustments.

As Blaine said, he doesn't have the disease, but he lives with it twenty-four hours a day. If the person with Parkinson's has a bad night, so does the caregiver. Caregivers seem to program themselves to awaken to any movements in their beds that are out of the ordinary. Blaine wakes up every time I get up to go to the bathroom, even though I may not need any help—just to make sure I'm all right.

When Blaine and I both worked, he helped with the housework responsibilities. Now he has assumed more of these chores. They are not entirely new to him, but what is new is his having to do my share as well.

I still help with putting away the laundry and with meal preparation. Also, we still shop for groceries and other things together. But when I buy new clothing, Blaine has to go into the fitting room to help me dress and undress. It's interesting to see the looks he gets sometimes when he tells the attendant that I have Parkinson's and need his help in the fitting room.

Blaine doesn't work away from home much anymore, because I have developed a problem of falling. In fact, when we returned home from our winter trip to Florida, we decided to subscribe to a Lifeline program. Now, if I fall and he's not around, I'm wearing a medallion that I can press. The program calls his pager, as well as emergency numbers for two other people to be alerted if he doesn't respond to the page.

Our church has set up programs with volunteers to provide transportation if someone needs it or to come to the house to help. Recently, we chose to use this service to help us out when Blaine had to spend a few hours in town for business.

I have two friends in particular who stop by frequently. We go out and do things together as well, and that also gives Blaine a break. Our children are concerned about the demands of caregiving on Blaine and try to make sure that he gets away from the house so that he'll stay healthy, both physically and mentally.

Still, Blaine asks me to go with him every time, and this helps me to get out even more. (As you can see, I'm not a shut-in, by any means!)

When the husband is the one with Parkinson's, however, and is larger physically than the wife, physical caregiving becomes more difficult.

One couple in our support group had an interesting problem because he is a large man, and his wife is an average-sized woman. On several occasions, electric power outages occurred while he was in his electric-lift chair, in a reclining position. It was quite a problem to get him out of the reclined chair, but like a lot of couples, they laughed about it and didn't make it a big issue.

Another wife of a man with Parkinson's, who has since passed away, said that her biggest problem was always being tired. This remark is common among caregivers with whom we have talked.

Sometimes the caregiver must take over the responsibilities of running the household, from paying bills to taking care of insurance and income taxes, to making other financial decisions the spouse had made before Parkinson's intruded into their lives.

Other new responsibilities may be deciding which home repairs to make and who should make them, or whether to replace old appliances or trade in an automobile. As the caregiver, the wife may now find that she has to learn to unplug a sink or a toilet, fix a sticking window, or do other things that her husband had always done.

One thing a person with Parkinson's needs to take responsibility for is not getting into impossible situations. One man with Parkinson's decided to do something on the roof, but once he got up there, he couldn't get down. There was no way his wife could help him.

In my case, I'm prone to falling. I learned that I'm likely to fall if I try to pick up something on the floor that I used to be able to retrieve easily. Now, I try to keep myself out of situations that will contribute to my falling. I leave the object there and ask Blaine to retrieve it when I need it. The more I do to keep myself in control, the less strain it will put on my caregiver.

Remember, if you are a martyr and complain all the time, it won't contribute to a good relationship with your caregiver. Blaine is familiar with all of my problems by now, and he doesn't need a continual barrage of my complaints.

Wearing a smile will take you a lot farther than a grumble or a frown. Smiling and laughing are contagious, and they will bear fruit down the road. It is also important for the caregiver to stay positive and happy, for the good health of both partners.

One thing that helps is for others to visit and extend their support. Our son is busy with his life of work, marriage, fathering two teenagers, involvement in church, and other activities, but he finds time to stop by about every other evening. The visits of our daughter (who lives a little farther away), our daughter-in-law, and our grandchildren are also very important. They may not know what a boost they give to me and Blaine, but sharing these times makes us realize that we are not alone.

It's important for caregivers to take time for themselves. Doing so will help them to stay healthy and keep their caregiving responsibilities in perspective. It will also prevent them from feeling trapped. For example, my mother needed constant care at the end of her illness. My sister found it a welcome relief to have a health-care aide come in every day for four hours to help with our mother.

Sometimes caregivers lash out at the ones they love when one of them has an illness. Partly, it may be because the caregiver feels trapped and can no longer come and go with the freedom of the past. All the caregivers whom I have talked to suffer from sleep deprivation, as well. The caregiver is always tired and edgy, so little things set off the nerves.

Caregivers feel the frustration of always having to wait for the person with Parkinson's, as well as the aggravation of cleaning up food spills each time the person eats and handling the additional laundry these mishaps create.

And, of course, it's simply difficult and fatiguing for caregivers to see their once healthy, vivacious partners now struggling with everything they do.

Caregivers often lack time and energy for once-enjoyed activities, not to mention that they have to worry about whether there will be enough money to take care of expenses.

The future, with all its uncertainties, is also frightening.

If the person with Parkinson's is married, the spouse will probably end up being the primary caregiver, but that role can be filled in a variety of ways, depending on the individual situation.

The caregiver may be one, or more, of the children. In other situations, perhaps a brother or a sister has taken on the responsibility. In still others, special friends have become caregivers.

And for people who have none of the above, there may be a paid person who comes to live in the home as the primary caregiver. In *any* situation, the caregiver can always use *some* help!

Professional help can come from public health services, visiting nurses, home health care, physical and occupational therapy, agencies on aging, adult day care, support groups, civic organizations, and churches. Check into these resources in your area.

Over the years, Blaine and I have found little ways to adjust to the invasion of Parkinson's into our marriage and our lives. We have found that we both need to put forth an effort to make life as pleasant and easy as possible.

To people with Parkinson's, we offer these suggestions:

- Learn to pace yourself. Overdoing makes the symptoms worse.
- Be optimistic. Smile. No one wants a sourpuss around.
- Be responsible for taking medication, noting any changes, and reporting them to your doctor.
- Allow extra time to get ready to go out. Try not to get flustered.
- Be responsible for getting exercise.
- Thank your spouse and let him know how much you appreciate him (or her).
- Give your spouse time to adjust to the new realities in your life together.
- Let your spouse know your needs and your feelings. (Blaine says, "I'm not a mind reader!")
- Communicate your needs pleasantly, without giving orders.
- Don't make yourself and everyone else miserable by frequently comparing yourself as you are now with the way you were before Parkinson's.
- Stay as active as possible. Don't give up.
- Educate yourself. Read everything you can find about Parkinson's.

To spouses (and other caregivers), Blaine offers these suggestions:

- Put extra medication in the car.
- Keep the car in good condition and filled with gas.
- Let your spouse off at the door of a store and then park.
- Be willing to change your lifestyle gradually.
- Do special things together, such as going out for Sunday morning breakfast.
- Allow extra time for activities.
- Develop patience. Leave the room if you become impatient with your partner's slowness.

- Don't be *too* helpful. Your partner needs activity and exercise.
- Don't be overprotective. Encourage independence.
- Involve your partner in as much of the family decision making as possible.
- Be alert to your partner's "on-off" times.
- Take one day at a time.
- Watch for changes in symptoms. Discuss them with your partner and the doctor.
- Don't smother the patient with worry.
- Encourage, praise, sympathize, but don't exaggerate.
- Be generous with your hugs.
- Encourage your partner to communicate his or her needs. Explain that you are not a mind reader.
- Be aware of your partner's emotional needs.
- Join a Parkinson's support group.
- Remember that even under the most perfect of circumstances, things don't always go smoothly. Do the best you can, which is all anyone can do.

CHAPTER 10

Relationships with Our Adult Children

You may give them your love but not your thoughts,
For they have their own thoughts.
You may house their bodies, but not their souls,
For their souls dwell in the house of tomorrow which you
    cannot visit. . . .
You are the bows from which your children as living arrows
    are sent forth.

—*Kahlil Gibran*

Whenever I am ill, even at my age, the person I still yearn for is my mother. She is the one who could always make me feel better, just by the touch of her hand, the way she expressed her concern, and the special things she cooked; she is the one who truly pampered me. I remember the special meal that Mom would make many years ago for her children when they were ill: homemade bread, toasted on the black woodstove (our only toaster), and covered with butter and cream. When one of her children was hurting, she would say, "If I could bear the pain for you, I would."

Now in her eighties, as I write this, she is no longer well, and I want so much to make her well or bear her pain for her. But I know that my tending isn't what she wants. She wants *her* Mama. Sometimes when I visit, she will say so: "I miss Mama," or "I feel as though Mama is here with me sometimes." She yearns for her mother, but with great determination she continues to mother me as I cope with my Parkinson's. And so the cycle continues.

Putting my mother, myself, and my children into perspective is important as I try to understand what is happening between me and my children since Parkinson's entered our lives. When I think about my mother's role in my life, I can begin to understand my children as they adjust to the invasion of an incurable disease into my life.

This chapter centers around my children, Susan and Randy, and their spouses, and how they have adjusted to their mother having Parkinson's disease. I hope it will help other parents to understand their children's reactions a little better.

It seems only a short while ago that Randy and Susan were children, playing ball, playing in the snow with neighborhood kids, or swimming with their friends in our backyard pool. It seems only a short while ago that the children camped with us on summer weekends or snowshoed with us in the winter in the snowy woods behind the house, where we built a fire and toasted frankfurters.

Susan, my elder child, was always serious and demanded a great deal of herself. She was also good, sweet, and thoughtful. She loved her dolls and toys, which she kept neat and well-organized. She enjoyed sewing and crafts, took dancing and piano lessons, and liked outdoor life, too. Although for some reason she doubted it, she was everything a daughter could be. I have always been proud of her accomplishments. She graduated from the University of Maine at Orono with a degree in Health and Family Life and then went back for additional study in early childhood education so that she could teach elementary school.

Susan married Keith in 1975, and they have two lovely children, Bethany and Elissa. Susan teaches kindergarten part-time, which lets her spend time with her children and be involved in their activities. She also has many interests and talents of her own.

When she and Keith bought an older home in Winterport, Susan took an active role in the remodeling and the redecorating. She takes advantage of workshop opportunities on such varied topics as education, dried-flower arrangements, and herbs. Susan is an excellent organizer. She enjoys collecting children's books and dreams of having her own bookstore one day. Winterport is fifteen miles from us, so we don't see Susan every day, but we telephone each other about three times a week.

Susan's husband, Keith, is very close to the family. In 1988, after ten years of success and stress in the world of big business, Keith brought his business expertise to become a copartner with Blaine and Randy in Atwood Builders. Keith has special interests in sailing, canoeing, and camping. He also enjoys attending theater and sports events with Susan. Most of all, doing things as a family is important to both Keith and Susan: one of their favorite activities is spending the day with the children on the Maine coast.

Randy, my younger child, was happy-go-lucky, affectionate, loving, and compassionate growing up. He was also independent and happy to entertain himself with his toys. Although he teased at times, he seldom fought or argued with anyone in the family or among his friends. He loved the outdoors and all the activities of the outdoorsman, and he still does—especially canoeing, fishing, and hunting.

After graduation, Randy's first career interest was farming, an interest that began during many childhood visits to his grandparents in northern Maine. Next door to his grandparents lived my brother, George, who had a potato farm and dairy cows. Randy loved and looked up to George and spent as much time as he could on the farm. We were not surprised when he chose to spend summers helping on the farm during his late teens.

While growing up, Randy was also exposed to woodworking and carpentry. He had watched Blaine work on many carpentry projects. Many of the carpenters in Blaine's family, like Blaine's father (who lived down the road from us), were furniture makers. Always creative, Randy appreciated their art, and as time passed, he, too, was drawn to carpentry. In 1983, when Blaine retired from teaching, Randy and Blaine formed the partnership of Atwood Builders. Randy brings a great deal of creative energy to his job, along with the warm personality that he has retained through the years.

In 1977, Randy married Debbie. Now they live a few steps down the street from us and have two beautiful children, Ashley and Joshua.

Debbie is a radiological technician at Eastern Maine Medical Center; now part-time, she has limited her hours since the arrival of the children. She enjoys her involvement in the children's activities, such as volunteering at their school, leading a Brownie troop, and teaching Sunday school. She is talented in crafts, especially basketmaking, knitting, and home decorating. Debbie and Randy are both very family oriented, and they enjoy the companionship of many other families who have the same interests. Because they live on our street, we see them very often.

When we first told the children (in 1981) that I had Parkinson's, I could see that the dominant emotion among the many they experienced was fear. They feared for me and feared for themselves. They made it clear that they would be here for me but that I would have to let them know what my needs were, because they knew so little about Parkinson's disease.

Because of the close relationship we have with our children, and because I know that true understanding comes from the openness of all parties, I had assumed that the children and I would talk freely about Parkinson's and what it was doing to me and to them. Over the years, that hasn't been the case. Why not? I'm not sure. Perhaps it's just been easier for each of us to avoid unpleasant topics. Perhaps I resist admitting that there are changes in me.

I've thought about what I want from the children and have discovered that it's not easy to know. I know that I do want a little sympathy, but I don't want pity. I want them to understand what I'm experiencing, yet I rarely explain to them what I experience. (I can explain more readily to strangers!) I want a word of praise to tell me they know how hard I'm trying, yet I rarely let them know how hard I'm trying. I want them to understand my limitations, but I don't tell them my limitations because I'm afraid they will impose further limitations on me.

For example, I fear limitations imposed on my time with my grandchildren. Once, I promised my four grandchildren that starting with the eldest, I would have each one in turn stay overnight during the next four nights. Immediately, my daughter and my daughter-in-law said to the children, "Now, don't get your hopes up, because that might be too much for Grandma." I explained to my grandchildren that I would not have asked them if I thought it might be too much for me. Still, when the fourth evening came, the youngest child trudged in with her little overnight bag, saying, "I thought I'd never get my turn; Mama said you'd be too tired." (I take advantage of opportunities to be with the grandchildren while they are small because they grow up so fast. Isn't it better to become tired interacting with children than to become bored resting alone?)

Over time, I've come to realize that the people with whom I find it hardest to talk about my Parkinson's are my mother and my children, although they are among the people I love best. Somehow, I think that the bond between mother and child is so deeply rooted in our emotions that we fear to discuss openly anything that threatens that bond. Possibly, I also fear that in discussing my Parkinson's with my children, I may damage their image of me as the capable, happy mother. Down deep, I fear that they will think less of me. So on both good days and bad days, I put on my best front and say, "Everything is fine." Mom, Susan, and Randy accept that without further probing because that's what they want to hear. This fear of communicating openly with them is a problem on which I continue to work. In the meantime,

I'll take Randy's advice: "Don't ignore your Parkinson's, and don't talk about it all the time either." In other words, find a balance.

To find a balance, both parent and child should speak openly from time to time. A word of praise or an expression of concern from the children lets the parent know that they are noticing things and they care. An expression of gratitude from the parent and sharing some of the parent's ups and downs lets the child know that he or she is an important part of the parent's world. Sometimes, sharing a good article on Parkinson's from a current newsletter can result in a productive discussion. Probably one of the best approaches is for the family to sit down periodically and discuss the situation. Sometimes each member can write his or her thoughts on paper for the others to read.

I have asked each of my children and their spouses to put their thoughts on paper for this chapter. I suggested that they comment on such things as their first reactions upon hearing my diagnosis, their views of the effect it has had on our family life, and any advice they would like to give to the families of people with Parkinson's. This exercise proved more useful than I antici-pated it might be: it showed me that the children still had some misconceptions about Parkinson's disease that I needed to discuss with them, such as Keith's idea that the more vigorously one exer-cises, the more one slows down the progression of the disease! It also showed me that Susan was still working her way through the four natural phases of grieving that most people experience when great loss, illness, or death enters their lives (disbelief or denial, anger, mourning, and acceptance). People spend various lengths of time on different stages: one person may whiz through all four stages, while another may spend a long time in one or more of them. Also, a person who has worked through these stages may find that he or she has reverted back to one of them, such as anger, because something in life has triggered it again. Learning how to deal with such a reversion is important, so that it doesn't lead to depression. Responding to what the children wrote, I overcame some of my reluctance to speak, and we had some productive breakthroughs in communication.

These were Randy's thoughts:

When I learned you had Parkinson's my first thoughts were questions: How far had it progressed? How far would it progress? What would help? Could it be passed on? The diagnosis of Parkinson's was upsetting, but your makeup and attitude were a big help.

When I come to your home, I see you up and around, so I am not reminded often that you have Parkinson's. I know you have days when you're tired. I've seen you when your medicine hasn't "kicked in." But the important thing to me is that you are still active—maybe not as active as you would have been—but I'm thankful that you get around as well as you do.

I guess my biggest fear is that the disease will progress, that you may become bedridden. I don't want to seem unconcerned about the stage you are in now, because I'm certainly not. We just do not usually see you at your worst.

I have thought several times how easy it would be for you to let yourself wallow in self-pity and not get out there and do the things you do. You are a real trooper, a champ! I can see how hard it is for you to do some of the things you do. You are the kind of person who thinks, "I can be miserable, or I can put forth some effort and do something." I give you a lot of credit for that.

I worry sometimes. We might be sitting at the table talking, and I will see your hand twitch, and that worries me. I think talking about our fears would help. I would be the first one to admit we just don't sit down and talk enough, and I probably don't express my feelings enough to you. There seems to be less time for long talks. I am married. I have my family responsibilities. It's a fact of life.

As for your relationship with the grandchildren, I don't think your Parkinson's has been a problem in any big way. Obviously, there are times when you might have to say, "I am sorry. I just don't feel up to playing with you today." Deb and I say the same thing. If we know you have been extra busy, we will say, "Grandma may be tired, so stay only half an hour." The children accept that because it has been that way from the beginning for them. We really appreciate what you do with them.

If I were to give advice to newly diagnosed parkinsonians, I would suggest that they remember that their adult children are busy with their own lives, but that does not mean that they don't care. Don't feel too resentful if you don't get all the support you would like from your children, and don't let resentment build up too long. Find some tactful way to let your children know how you are feeling.

I would advise the adult children of parkinsonians to explain to their parents that they want to take a positive approach. Let's not ignore the Parkinson's; let's talk if someone wants to talk. Let's do things together.

These were Debbie's thoughts:

At the time I learned about your Parkinson's, I was preoccupied with Ashley. I was really involved with pregnancy, babies, and motherhood. Here I was with this new baby, and my first concern was for her and her well-being. So the first thing I worried about was whether Parkinson's is hereditary. I remember looking up what information I could find about Parkinson's and calming my fears that way.

I think your Parkinson's has affected our family life in positive ways. Your retirement from teaching has enabled you to spend so much time with our children. I think that your awareness that sometime down the road you may not have the stamina to do all you would like to do with them spurs you on to do all you can now. I feel fortunate that you take time to do so many things for the children. Many people procrastinate and say, "I will do it tomorrow." You do a lot of fun things today. Like the day you took the children, along with four of the neighbor's children, to make old-fashioned May baskets. They will always have those times to remember. You do a terrific job with the children.

I remember one thing that used to worry me at the beginning, before you were on medication. I had read that it was important to let the patient do most things for himself to keep himself flexible. I would see people coddling you. I would see Blaine doing things like getting you an electric toothbrush because it was difficult for you to coordinate brushing your teeth. I would see Susan writing out a check for you instead of making you push yourself to do it. I thought, "Keep it up, and you will have her in a wheelchair." I know if I were the one with Parkinson's, I would want to be pampered. I would be feeling sorry for myself. So I was afraid you would give up and let your Parkinson's progress faster. After you started taking medication, I was encouraged when you were so improved, and I could see you were not giving up.

I know Parkinson's is a slowly progressing disease, but when I see parkinsonians at the hospital who have progressed much further than you have, it really upsets me because I think that some day you may be in that same situation.

It is not easy to think about your Parkinson's progressing. It has appeared to remain stable for several years, and we have been comfortable with the way you are. We know that you do get tired, that you have "ons" and "offs," and that you have some difficulty with such things as fastening a seat belt. Those changes have been so gradual that we have become used to them and barely see them. That makes it harder when we do notice a change. For example, I have begun to notice how your foot is twisting at times. The first time I saw your foot moving that way, I was startled and thought, "No, she is not supposed to be doing that!" Changes are scary.

All four of us go through spells of feeling guilty because we don't do more or don't take enough time to listen to you. It's difficult to find time to fit everything in. There is so much going on in our lives. But when we do sit down and talk with you, and let you get your feelings out, we feel better. For us, it is important to know what is going on with you.

These were Susan's thoughts:

I remember when you first voiced your concern about the weakness and shaking in your hand when you were trying to write letters to me. I didn't think you were serious. I laughed and joked that you were trying to get out of writing to me. The thought was totally unexpected that you would ever change or that something would come into our lives that could affect us so adversely.

When you were finally diagnosed, I was shocked, confused, and upset. I didn't want the doctors to find anything. I wanted everything to be fine and to stay as it was. After the initial shock, I was both confused and concerned. I had so many questions but was almost afraid to ask them for fear of what the answers would be. I was concerned for you and what this meant for you. Where were you now in this progressive disease, and where would you go?

Then I felt another wave of shock and the misapprehension that Parkinson's disease could affect my baby and my future children. I was really frightened. Could this disease take over my children's bodies and my own as well? In the days and weeks that followed, I wanted to learn as much as I could about it, and I wanted you to do the same. I think I was hoping to find a way to get it out of our lives. I had moved from confusion to anger that this was happening to us.

Then I got tired of hearing about Parkinson's and just wanted to forget about it. I realize I was very selfish and often I still am. Maybe I felt the Parkinson's threatening the closeness we had always shared, slowly building a wall between us. Or am I myself building the wall? I am not sure. I resent the Parkinson's, and the resentment spills over. I wanted our relationship to remain the way it was. I miss all the things we used to do and all the laughter. I fear a possible role reversal, for which I may not ever be strong enough.

My feelings are often in turmoil about you: love, fear, resentment, anger, and guilt. I know that I don't always meet your needs. My own family and work take so much of my time now. But I want you to know that I am proud of you, proud that you have continued your teaching role in forming the support group, that you are writing this book, that you continue to reach out to people, and that you continue to enjoy meeting new faces and seeing new places.

These are Keith's thoughts:

My first reaction to the news of your Parkinson's was one of confusion because I didn't know much about the disease. After hearing more about Parkinson's, I felt sorrow for you and concern about the rate at which the disease might progress. I also began to be concerned that Parkinson's might be hereditary. How might it affect my wife and children? I still have questions in that area.

Over the years, I think everyone has handled things reasonably well. Maybe we could have encouraged you to exercise more vigorously to slow down the progression of the disease. Often I was frustrated because you did not react in the same way as I would have reacted. I have since learned that you are doing what is right for you. You have done a super job of increasing your understanding of the disease.

My advice to any children of parents newly diagnosed is to educate yourself as much as possible about Parkinson's disease and to allow your parents as much latitude as possible to determine, with the doctor, the best course of treatment for them. The most important job of the children is to provide whatever support they can.

In reading these messages from my children and their spouses, you can see how many conflicting, and even overwhelming, feelings are generated when Parkinson's enters the life of the family. How should the parents react to these feelings? Keep the lines of communication open. Be patient. Help to educate the children. Give or lend them a copy of this book and other recent publications on Parkinson's. Ask the major Parkinson's organizations to put your children on their mailing lists for newsletters and other informative literature. Ask your children to attend support group meetings with you from time to time. Maintain a positive attitude.

I've had only brief contact with the adult children of other people with Parkinson's, but I'll share with you something I've observed:

Every once in a while, adult daughters appear at our support group meetings or call me on the telephone. Often they are torn apart because one parent has Parkinson's and the other parent cannot accept it. Sometimes the daughter lives a substantial distance from the parents. Why do the daughters, and not the sons, come to meetings or call on the phone? I don't know. But be prepared for the probability that your daughter will be more actively involved in assisting you than your son is.

Of course, many adult children are caregivers when the person with Parkinson's has no spouse. Much of what I have said about spouses (in the last chapter) applies to adult children who are the principal caregivers. However, even more than the spouse, the adult child needs a life of his or her own. One woman and her elderly mother with Parkinson's attended our support group meetings for five years. The daughter, who lived with her mother, brought her to every meeting, even after the mother was confined to a wheelchair. The mother, despite her infirmity, was always so cheerful and positive. Perhaps employing a paid, part-time caregiver helped the mother–daughter relationship. The daughter had time to pursue her own interests, and the mother had no guilt feelings that might have resulted from consuming all of her daughter's time and energy. If a caregiver submerges too much of herself or himself in the care of a loved one, feelings of anger and resentment are bound to surface, and no one will be happy. If a paid attendant is out of financial reach, other relatives could be asked to assist with time or with some of the money needed to pay for a part-time attendant.

Sometimes adult children live at a great distance from their parents in another part of the state or the country. No matter where the children live, it's important for them to communicate regularly, to visit, and to have their parents as guests if possible. Letters, phone calls, and little gifts help to keep up morale and help to maintain the good attitude that is so important to the well-being of a person with Parkinson's. Children can look through a medical supply store for little things that will make the parent's life easier. One busy man was surprised and delighted, for example, when his daughter gave him a small pocket pillbox with a built-in timer. This thoughtful little gift enables him to take his medications on time as he moves from activity to activity.

The person with Parkinson's will experience a quicker emotional recovery if a sense of caring and support is extended by the children. At the same time, it's important for adult children to refrain from pushing their advice too assertively on the parent who has Parkinson's. Sometimes the advice is taken as criticism. According to a study by Dr. Shelley E. Taylor and Dr. Gayle Dakof of California, family members can best help a patient by showing concern and affection. They can be encouraging about the patient's ability to cope. But advice is taken better when it comes from doctors, other medical personnel, or other patients going through the same circumstances (see *The Journal of Personality and Social Psychology*, February 1990). According to Dr. Taylor, there is also a delicate balance between showing too much and too little concern about a patient's condition. "If you show too much concern, you'll seem to be catastrophizing, making it even worse than it is. If you accept the problem too calmly, you seem to be trivializing it."

In addition to caring for the parent with Parkinson's, the adult child must remember the other parent, too—the one who doesn't have Parkinson's disease. It's just as important for the children to be sensitive to his or her needs. Both parents' lives have changed, and they both need support and understanding.

What is the best advice for all family members? Be attentive, caring, and supportive of each other; keep the lines of communication open; and educate yourselves as much as possible about Parkinson's disease.

CHAPTER 11

Out of the Mouths of Babes . . .

I love you forever
I like you for always
As long as I'm living
My baby you'll be.

—Robert Munsch

It's ironic that grandparenthood and Parkinson's disease entered my life at the same time. In 1980, the first two of my grandchildren were born, and in the same year, my Parkinson's manifested itself. The arrival of grandchildren brought pure delight; the arrival of Parkinson's brought frustration and sorrow. When the time came to share the news, I received two very different messages: Shout from the rooftops that you are a grandmother; keep quiet about the Parkinson's.

Everyone knew how much I had looked forward to being a grandmother, and soon they knew that I had attained that status. But I made up my mind very quickly to be open about my Parkinson's, too. Especially with my grandchildren. I had no wish for secrecy about it.

This chapter is about another of life's most fulfilling relationships, the bond with one's grandchildren. It's about the grandparent's need to develop and enjoy that relationship, as well as to be open and honest with the grandchildren about Parkinson's.

Many people avoid discussing serious problems with children, problems such as an illness, a death in the family, or a change in family circumstances. They fear upsetting the children and, in a mistaken desire to protect them, delay such discussions "until the children are older." In some of these instances, I believe the adults may really be protecting themselves from facing things that they themselves fear.

Today most psychologists support my position that children need to be told the truth (in an appropriate way) about circumstances that arise. It's easier to teach children positive attitudes in their early years than to change their attitudes when they are older. And it's better to prevent the misinterpretations that develop when discussion is avoided. Children sense when something is being kept from them, and they are likely to build up in their minds whatever they imagine.

When children sense that there is a problem, they need to be reassured. In a recent instance, a seven-year-old whom we know was found crying while the adults in his family mourned the loss of a relative. The boy barely knew the deceased man. When asked why he was crying, he said that he didn't like to see everybody so sad. When he received assurance that this was a normal part of the process of grieving and saying good-bye, he was content to go off and play.

A grandparent's Parkinson's is impossible to hide. When adults avoid the subject, children may begin to believe that something about the grandparent is so bad that it must not be talked about. Don't be afraid to talk with your grandchildren and let them express their fears, which will help them adjust to your Parkinson's.

My conviction about helping children to express their fears comes from my own childhood experience with fears, especially the fear of dying. I believe that this fear was caused by the deaths of people close to me, which no one discussed with me or helped me to accept. When I was three, my aunt, only in her thirties, died of pneumonia, and soon afterward, my grandfather Wotton died. I was young, but I still recall a roomful of sad people. When I was seven, another aunt, who lived just across the road, died, followed in a month by my uncle. They left three children who were split up among the relatives. The youngest, my age, came to live with us. With the deaths of so many relatives, I developed many fears, because no one had ever discussed death or the facts about these deaths with me. Because these events were never open to discussion, I never expressed my fears, nor did I receive the reassurance I needed.

Not all children are so reticent about exploring the subjects of their fears. Eight-year-old Johnny is one of those exceptions. But his story, too, illustrates the child's need for explanation and reassurance. Johnny lives in Vermont, and his grandparents, people we know, live in Maine. Whenever he visits Maine, he has a wonderful time with them and all of his cousins. On one visit, his grandfather, who had Parkinson's, was experiencing a serious problem with dyskinesia (involuntary movements). Johnny became very upset. He demanded to know what was wrong, and, in response to explanations, why no one had told him! Johnny's response was a healthy one. He wanted openness.

Any changes in a child's life need to be made as painless as possible, whether they involve his or her parents' divorce, a relative's death, or a grandparent's Parkinson's. Your grandchild should be told that you aren't going to die from Parkinson's. It's helpful to explain—in as positive a way as possible—what Parkinson's means to you and your family. You can make the child feel important and needed.

In talking with other families in which a member had Parkinson's, I learned that many adults would answer a child's question but wouldn't bring up the subject of Parkinson's themselves. Yet opening the subject up to discussion is really the adult's responsibility.

We know that young children tend to be very accepting of situations in which they find themselves. Many children are born into families that are coping with one problem or another, and they accept the problem as a familiar fact of life. The problems of Parkinson's can become one of those familiar facts of life for the child. It's expected that Grandpa takes a long time to shave, just as Billy takes a long time to tie his shoes, and Billy understands. Perhaps Billy has to give Grandpa a hand to help him out of a chair, just as there are many things that Grandpa does for Billy. Of course, the attitude of the whole family influences the child's attitude toward the person who has Parkinson's. Billy's attitude will be a good one if the family thinks of every member as a blessing and not a burden.

Let your grandchildren be as much a part of your life as they would have been if you had not had Parkinson's. They will appreciate having someone with whom to play a game of checkers, take a walk, or just talk.

Grandparents are an important part of the growing child's life. With openness, the grandparent's limitations become known, accepted, and even expected. But sometimes the child can be happily surprised, as was Chris, the grandson of a man with Parkinson's whom we know.

When Chris was born, Gramp had already had Parkinson's for several years, and when Chris was five, Gramp retired. Chris was very happy about all the time his grandfather spent with him. Gramp taught him how to ride a bicycle and how to skate and shared many other activities with him. Gramp's slowness didn't bother Chris, although every once in a while Chris needed to be reassured that Gramp was "all right." He had come to expect Gramp's slowness. One day, Gramp proposed that they play a game of hockey, and they put on their skates. Pleased, because being with Gramp was always fun, Chris (now seven) expected a good but slow game. However, on this day, Gramp's medication, attitude, and skating rhythm all worked together perfectly, and he surprised everyone by playing a fast, exciting game. Imagine the boy's delight! I have the feeling that Chris will carry the memory of that game for a long time.

Young children's easy acceptance of problems is not necessarily true of teenagers. Teens are often reluctant to face and talk about family members' problems. I've talked to a number of grandparents with Parkinson's who have similar stories. Their teenage grandchildren behave as if they're unaware of a problem, but they're obviously concerned. One grandmother's observation is typical: her grandson seemed to be unsure of just how to handle the subject of her Parkinson's and didn't ask any questions. Nevertheless, he was anxious to help, promptly opening doors, extending a hand to help her up from her chair, bringing items she needed. Because teenagers are reluctant to ask questions (perhaps out of fear of intruding or prying), they would probably appreciate their grandparents' initiative in opening a discussion about Parkinson's and encouraging them to ask questions. Perhaps a good starting point for a discussion would be a gift to your teenage grandchild of the book *When Bad Things Happen to Good People*, by Harold S. Kushner. Or perhaps no starting point is needed, just a straightforward discussion. Teenagers love their grandparents, and they deserve information, so that they know where things stand.

Some teens reach out to help in very meaningful ways. Eighteen-year-old Ellen Levin loved her grandfather Abe Brickman, who had Parkinson's, very much. She helped her mother organize a PEP (Parkinson's Educational Program) support group in her home city of St. Louis, and she wrote a very moving piece called "Mirror, Mirror on the Wall," published by PEP-USA in California (see the excerpt in chapter 6).

I'd like you to meet my grandchildren and share some of my experiences with them when they were young children.

Ashley is the eldest. The daughter of Randy and Debbie, she was born in Maine in the spring of 1980, with blond hair and huge blue eyes. She is everything a grandma could hope for. One has only to look into those large eyes to see the love and caring within. As the eldest, she is the leader of the pack, over the occasional objections of the others.

Bethany, the daughter of Susan and Keith, arrived in the fall of 1980. I flew to Wisconsin to welcome this little replica of her mother. As special as my first grandchild, Bethany is a deep thinker and very observing.

Joshua, the brother of Ashley, arrived with a twinkle in his eyes on St. Patrick's Day, 1982. He is a loving, happy child and a tease. He is very pleased with himself for being the only grandson!

The youngest grandchild, Elissa, was born in the spring of 1983 in Vermont, where I went to welcome her and help with her sister, Bethany. Elissa has always been perpetual motion. She flies into my arms as she yells "Grandma!" and she chooses the most unexpected times to run up and hug me or gently kiss the back of my hand.

What happiness these children bring me!

I had always looked forward to being the best grandma ever, at least in my grandchildren's eyes. When my year-long symptoms were first diagnosed as Parkinson's disease, I was afraid that the disease would prevent me from being the type of grandparent I wished to be. At the same time, I knew that Blaine and I had a great deal of love to give our grandchildren, and I felt that we could contribute a great deal to their lives.

By the time I was diagnosed, Ashley was a year old. I decided to start using the word *Parkinson's* when I was with her. For example, I might say, "My hands are so clumsy! If I didn't have Parkinson's, I could do a better job on this diaper." This wasn't for her benefit at that young age but for mine. I needed to get used to saying the word comfortably when I was around her. By the time she was two, she could explain that Grandma needed help sometimes because she had Parkinson's. Without being asked, she could help me pull a sweater down in the back. This was something special that she could do for me.

I have used the same approach with the other grandchildren, who have also had the benefit of the older ones' examples to follow. They understand what they need to know about my Parkinson's, and they help. They even see me cry on occasion (very infrequently), and they hug me and bring back my smile.

Once when Elissa was two, Susan and her children were visiting, and I became so frustrated at my limitations that I felt tears welling up in my eyes. I slipped away to my bedroom, and, face-down on the bed, I let myself cry. Before long, I heard little footsteps and saw Elissa climb up on the bed. I'll never forget her loving touch as she reached over and, without words, began softly rubbing my back, somehow knowing that what comforted her would surely comfort Grandma.

On another occasion, when Ashley was four, I became very tired. I said, "It makes me so frustrated that I have to have Parkinson's." Ashley replied, "That's okay, Grandma, just as long as you don't think more about your Parkinson's than you do your grandchildren." It was just what I needed to get me thinking positively again.

As life goes on, the children are learning that Grandma is the person inside the body that just happens to have a tremor and just happens to be slowed down with Parkinson's. One day when Bethany was very young, she stared at my fingers, which were involved in a nice little tremor. Soon she started moving her fingers. "Look, Grandma," she said, "I can wiggle my fingers, just like you."

The children are in elementary school now and are quite comfortable talking about my Parkinson's. This conversation, for example, took place on the way to an outing:

> ASHLEY: We're lucky you have Parkinson's because we get to help you.
> ELISSA: We get to help you get things. We get to reach up in the cupboard for you.
> JOSHUA: Yes, and by helping you, we're learning how to help other people.
> BETHANY: And Mommy told us that some grandmas never play with their grandchildren.

ASHLEY: Josh and I are lucky. We can just call and walk over any time, and if we are upset, we can talk it over with Grandma.
BETHANY: If you didn't have Parkinson's, you'd probably be working and so busy you'd hardly know us.
ASHLEY: And Grandma, you don't even look like you've got Parkinson's.

Bless their hearts!

Then to put the frosting on the cake, Ashley put a letter on my refrigerator door, which said,

Dear Grandma,
    You are the best Grandma in the world.
        Love,
        Ashley

Early in my Parkinson's, I knew that if I were to establish the kind of relationship I wanted with my grandchildren, I'd have to set priorities. I wouldn't be able to do everything I might want to do with the children and still have enough time for myself and Blaine. I examined my priorities. First, if I am to be a productive person, I must allow time for activities that will enrich my life and help me to grow. Second, I need to have time with Blaine. Third, I need to have time with my grandchildren.

When the grandchildren come to my house, they have my complete attention. The housework doesn't get done, but we have a real visit! I have a special place for games, books, toys, and dress-up clothes, and I keep a stock of paper, paints, scissors, and other supplies. But the two things the children enjoy most with me are having a tea party and having My Special Time with Grandma Day. A tea party is more fun than a snack, because a snack is merely eating. A tea party requires a table to be set decoratively, at least two people to be present, and interesting conversation to take place. My Special Time with Grandma Day is for one child at a time. Since Bethany and Elissa moved to Maine, it is not easy to be attentive to all four grandchildren at once. So the children sometimes take turns, and each one gets my undivided attention. Although they don't like waiting for their turns, they know the system is fair, and they know their turns are coming.

In the beginning I was afraid that Parkinson's would interfere with my relationship with my grandchildren. In fact, it has had little effect on that relationship. In some ways, it has brought us closer than if Parkinson's had not necessitated my retirement.

I want to close this chapter by sharing something that Joshua once wrote in school. The things that please me most about it are the positive feelings he obviously has about visiting our home and the fact that Parkinson's did not even rate a comment:

10/20/89

My Grandma

My Grandma lives just down the road. She is around 58. I like the activities she sets out for us to do. One of the activities I liked was the banner for our cousin's birthday.

Her real name is Glenna. She used to be a teacher.

Her husband is Blaine. He used to be a teacher, too. We call him Pa. I *love* his homemade ice cream.

My Grandma is *super* nice.

My grandchildren have taught me that children don't measure their grandparents' love or the good times they have with them by outward appearances or the speed with which they move. I see that if the adults in a child's life are happy and comfortable, the children will be also.

Our grandchildren are now young adults. They have grown up accepting Parkinson's as part of my life, and our love and relationships have not suffered because of it. An example of this is the time our granddaughter Ashley had to give a public speech on an outstanding person. She chose to write and deliver a speech about me and came in third in the public contest. Of course, I was very proud.

CHAPTER 12

One Day at a Time!

Look to this day!
For it is life, the very life of life.
In its brief course lie all the varieties and realities of your
    existence:
The bliss of growth;
The glory of action;
The splendor of beauty;
For yesterday is already a dream, and tomorrow is only
    a vision;
But today, well-lived, makes every yesterday
A dream of happiness, and every tomorrow a vision
    of hope.

—*From the Sanskrit*

"Today, well-lived . . ." What a meaningful phrase! Living well each day means dealing with life in the most positive manner our resources will allow. It may not bring happiness every hour or even every day. It may sometimes include having a good cry, the kind of brief release that enables us to get on with living. But making the most of each day is of utmost importance to people with Parkinson's: it gives us control over our lives and a sense of satisfaction and accomplishment. Best of all, while we are actively involved in pursuits that we care about, our symptoms often disappear! We are amazed at what we can accomplish!

A good way to reflect on our lives from day to day is to keep a diary or a journal and set aside time several days a week to make entries. The diary gives us a safe place to vent our frustrations, set goals, and record the daily successes we experience in our lives. Of course, we all have good days and bad days. When we can see all of our entries about good days, we can cope better with the bad days. When we reread entries about bad days, we realize that they are balanced by good days.

In this chapter, I'll share with you some of the entries in my journal. They extend from my earliest frustrating time with Parkinson's (before I began taking Sinemet) up to 1998. They give glimpses of my life with Parkinson's and also show how I used the journal to help me cope. Among the entries, I will intersperse excerpts from some letters written by Dr. Feldman, apprising my family doctor of my status; these excerpts will give you an objective look at my particular case of Parkinson's. (I will not include material about medications and dosages contained in Dr. Feldman's letters.)

January 1982—Today I am evaluating the progression of my Parkinson's symptoms. The only medication I've taken is Benadryl [given to me by Dr. Cross, my family physician], and that has been reduced because of the side effects of itchy, scratchy eyes and low blood count. The side effects have lessened, but the tremor in my right hand is more pronounced. When I eat, my spoon or fork is likely to jiggle. My lower lip trembles occasionally. I have more stiffness in my right hand and arm. Handwriting is slow and difficult. My right leg drags, and the pain in my right hip causes me to limp. I think that the pain may be caused by the fact that my right side is slower and more rigid than my left, and my body has difficulty synchronizing.

Dressing presents some problems, especially putting on pantyhose. After trying various methods, I find that the easiest way to get into pantyhose is to lie on my back with my leg up and pull the hose down, rather than up. How graceful can one get? Another problem is dressing quickly enough to be ready when Blaine wants to leave for school. He does help me, though, and he is patient.

At school, my main problem is fatigue. I look at my class, and I'm overwhelmed with the responsibility of teaching these teenagers. At home I can look at a task and decide whether or not I want to do it. I can't do that with a roomful of students.

Emotionally and mentally, I feel that I'm doing well. It's been almost a year since my Parkinson's was diagnosed, and although each morning I still have to adjust to the knowledge that I have Parkinson's, I rarely feel down. I get frustrated because of the limitations imposed by the Parkinson's, but I'll keep working at accepting the limitations. I'm determined to remain positive.

April 1983—DR. FELDMAN: Of the targets of therapy that one might look at are included mild rigidity involving both upper and lower extremities, reduced arm swing when walking, reduced eye-blink frequency, immobile posture, and decreased spontaneous shifts in sitting, difficulty in turning over in bed, difficulty in buttoning, difficulty with bimanual tasks, such as stirring, clapping hands; slowness of movements in general.

Mrs. Atwood has clearly used "mind over matter" to intentionally lift her legs higher than she feels they are being lifted in order to clear the ground. This conscious effort results in her ability to compensate for the rigidity, and the decrease and removal of associated movements that she has had. A mild tremor of her fingers exists, but this is no problem. She is able to run, and her arm swing is more normal when she runs. She is able to do things such as making applique, comforters, etc., but slowly. I feel that she could benefit from low-dose Sinemet.

[Note: This small amount of Sinemet did wonders for me. Some of my symptoms disappeared; others became milder.]

June 1983—Today I focused on the importance of doing a task or a project, rather than on the time it takes me to do it. I see that by pacing myself, I can accomplish a moderate amount each day.

I was reminded again of Blaine's mother [at eighty-seven] working on a square of patchwork for a quilt for Susan or Randy. She said, "If I get one square completed in each day, I feel I have accomplished something." One square of patchwork isn't much, but doing one each day enabled her to create a beautiful heirloom that will be used down through the generations.

I also thought about how nice it's been this past year to be retired and have more free time for myself. My job had taken up so much of my time for so long, I hadn't had time for other things I wanted to do. Now I give myself the luxury of time to please myself—I undertake projects that I want to undertake and spend more time with family and friends.

November 1983—Today I made my second trip to Boston Medical Center to see Dr. Feldman. He writes to Dr. Cross that "when she walks, there is a slight decrease in the arm swing on the right side, but she is able to get up out of a chair, her eyes are blinking, her face is soft with wrinkles, and she has no evidence of Parkinson's disease to the gross observation." The small doses of Sinemet have made a great improvement in my life.

January 1984—A day begins; I am half awake. I feel relaxed and I snuggle down, happy that I don't have to hop right out of bed. In no time, my hand begins to shake, just as if someone had thrown a switch and turned it on. Through conscious effort I finally get it under control. Next, the muscles in my right arm tighten up uncomfortably. I tell myself, "Okay, just relax. Exercise the arm a bit and go back to sleep." It is 5:15 A.M., and Blaine rolls out of bed, quietly picking up the clothes that he so thoughtfully laid out the night before. Now I will go back to sleep. Once more I turn over. Uh-oh. No easy task. All those years that I just flipped over automatically whenever I wanted to. . . . Now I have to think about it. I sit up in bed, reposition my hips, and, bit by bit, I get into my new position.

I'm still restless. I may as well get up. Only 6 A.M., but I've always been a morning person. Somehow it seems important to remind myself that Parkinson's hasn't affected me that much. Getting out of bed isn't difficult, but I feel like someone I don't know as I try to lift my feet to get to the bathroom and then the kitchen. "The early morning shuffle!"

When I reach the kitchen, I feel better. Finding Blaine there, sipping coffee and reading the paper, is reassuring. And I get the feeling he's glad I'm there, too. What a blessing that we have each other! Once more I am reminded that Parkinson's is just an inconvenience that we can handle. I have a cup of coffee with Blaine and take my medication. Blaine leaves.

After a leisurely look at the paper, I shower and get dressed. I've always liked wearing bright, pretty clothes, and dressing is one of my favorite times, although occasionally it's frustrating. I look in the mirror and pull my shoulders back. I'm ready to "look to this day!"

May 1984—Dr. FELDMAN: Her Parkinson's disease shows some rigidity in her right hand, but otherwise she has only bradykinesia to show. She has ability to do fine manipulations and her facial expression is excellent with no significant reduction in eyeblink frequency. The only problem she actually has is the feeling of a lack of power.

I would like her to exercise as much as possible and to stretch her arms and back; otherwise, she is in generally excellent condition and is doing very well.

July 1984—Today I cry! I know that frequent crying stems from depression, from unwillingness to accept one's situation, or from an attempt to manipulate people's feelings. But an occasional cry can be a positive force if it's used as a healthy outlet for pent-up feelings. Several articles I've read have said that crying may be a way of excreting chemical by-products of stress. Both men and women feel better after crying. Just yesterday [a friend] called and began to cry about something that affected her. After a while, she said, "I feel better now."

When I "cry on someone's shoulder," it's good to feel the other person's caring, especially if the person with the shoulder doesn't say, "Don't cry." But more often, like today, I cry alone. Crying alone has its advantages. I can let myself go and become as miserable as I please, counting off all the reasons to feel sorry for myself.

I'm crying today because I'm afraid. I'm convinced my Parkinson's is getting worse. I face a full-length mirror. Is that a little stoop I see? Is my face developing the Parkinson's mask? I cry because I feel out of control. Everywhere I look there's something to be done, and I have no energy to tackle it. The simplest tasks seem so monumental. I remember how I used to be able to do so much. I cry (big, monstrous sobs by now) because I hate being so slow, because my grandchildren will know me only as a slowpoke. (I know this is just an excuse for renewed sobbing.) I'm wallowing in misery.

My eyes are red and swollen, and I have a big pile of tissues proving that I needed this cry. But I seem to be running out of unhappy thoughts. Enough is enough! I hear the old refrain in my mind: "Many people in the world are in situations much worse than yours!" and I agree with it. It's time to get up, give thanks for all I've got and all I can still accomplish, and get on with living.

November 1984—Dr. FELDMAN: Glenna will begin to exercise and get rid of the stiffness between her shoulder blades, which is a tightness because of her posture. It is important for her to exercise her back muscles and avoid the flexed posture that one gets with Parkinson's, which is on the low side of treatment. Therefore, stretching of her limbs and stretching of her back, swimming, and just lying flat against gravity would be helpful. This should be done at the peak of her medication so that she can get the maximum stretch. Aerobic dance class would be excellent, because of the association of music and rhythm to automatic movements.

May 1985—Dr. FELDMAN: Glenna Atwood is doing extremely well on a small amount of Sinemet. . . . Exercise and activity will be continued, and I feel that most important is that Mrs. Atwood has a good attitude toward controlling her medications in a way that she finds benefit from them and utilizes the "power" as needed.

October 1985—Blaine and I have been traveling, and we pulled our RV into a campground. After setting up and enjoying our supper, we went for an evening walk. The fall air was crisp, ideal for walking. Soon we met a man and a woman, obviously a son and his mother, also out for a walk; the son held the mother's arm to steady her. We stopped and talked a bit.

Observing people is an interesting pastime. I saw that the mother had Parkinson's and that she was confused. She kept tugging at her son, urging him to come along. Nevertheless, all of the time, the man was very gentle and patient with his mother.

I reflected that the woman must have been a wonderful mother who taught her son love and respect by loving and respecting him. As I observed the frail, bent lady and her handsome, middle-aged son, I imagined a young mother chatting with a friend as her little boy tugged at her, urging her to come with him.

We continued our walk, feeling a sense of security. I had been reminded that I, too, have loved ones who will see me through, no matter what the future may bring.

October 1986—Today I am happy. Each day, I remember I have Parkinson's to deal with, and each day I make the deliberate choice to be happy in spite of my Parkinson's. So, I'm usually happy, but today I want to *think* about being happy.

Today I'm happy to be alive, to be able to laugh, to sing, to talk. I love to talk. I'm happy that I still have my voice!

I'm happy for all the good things—family, friends, and home—but I'm especially happy today because, as I look around our home, I see that it is full of wonderful memories.

I am not happy that I have Parkinson's, but I am happy that I've met so many wonderful people because of my Parkinson's. We gather together and support each other. I'm happy that I have a telephone so that other people with Parkinson's and their families can call me for information or just to talk. I'm happy that state health agencies refer them to me for information. I'm happy that I live in this age of medical research because of the medications that are now available. I'm bolstered in the hope that a cure for Parkinson's may be just ahead.

Today I'm happy because Randy stopped by to give me a hug. I'm happy because Ashley and Joshua came by to wait for the school bus. Blaine made breakfast for me. My friend invited me to her cottage by the lake.

When I get up in the morning, I can choose to be happy or sad. I prefer to be happy.

March 1987—Today I observed a gentleman at the grocery store. I could see by his stooped posture and masklike expression that he had Parkinson's disease. Somewhat detached from his surroundings, he pushed the grocery cart slowly, while his wife, shopping list in hand, flitted around, picking up groceries. He seemed almost unaware of her. I wondered what he was thinking. I decided that he wasn't too concerned about where she was in relation to him, since he knew she would come to him. Maybe just being there with each other was enough.

I reflected on the ability of people to adjust to what life brings them, the resiliency to adjust to things they never thought they'd have to adjust to. I thought about this man, who had probably been strong and hardworking at some former time, never picturing himself in this situation, with a spouse who never imagined it either. Yet here they were, carrying on with their lives. One does what one has to do.

June 1987—Today I'm thinking of the misconceptions that people have about illnesses and the way they attribute behavior they don't understand in others to an illness or a physical condition. I remember when Mom was middle-aged, every time she was nervous or felt unwell—or every time she opened the door to get some air—we'd roll our eyes and say, "It's her 'change of life.'" In my case, my Parkinson's gets the blame. I never heard anyone say that my behavior had anything to do with menopause. In fact, it almost seems as if menopause passed me right by. Whenever my behavior puzzled people, they said, "Well, she has Parkinson's, you know."

The assumptions that people make about Parkinson's bother me. When they say about a person with very advanced Parkinson's, "He's very feeble, but, you know, he still seems to have a good mind," they are assuming that a feeble body houses a feeble mind. No doubt they assume that one day *my* Parkinson's will lead to a feeble mind. Well, someday I *may* lose my mind, but probably not because of Parkinson's!

May 1988—Today Dr. Feldman rebalanced my medications because of the involuntary movements of my feet that I have experienced (a symptom of overmedication). With deprenyl [Eldepryl], apparently I need less Sinemet.

May 1988—Some time ago I received a call from a gentleman in Portland who had contacted a state health center to ask for information about Parkinson's disease and had been given my name and telephone number. The man's daughter, an eighth-grader named Jill, had read an article in the newspaper about Parkinson's and thought she might research that topic for her school's science fair. She needed more information. I was pleased to see a parent helping his child access information, and, like any ex-teacher, I was happy to help.

I sent Jill a packet of information (fortunately, there is much more information available today than there was when I first looked for it), and soon I received a nice "thank you" letter and a number of questions about my experience with Parkinson's: How long had I had Parkinson's disease? How had I adjusted to it? And how had it affected my life? We exchanged letters, and she pursued the topic.

Today I received a large envelope from my young friend. Inside was a copy of her report, the culmination of weeks of work, that she had gotten back from her teacher. I read it eagerly. It had received an "A."

August 1988—Today I almost drowned. I almost drowned despite my own safety rules about swimming: I must never swim alone; I must never swim until I have first tested my balance and coordination in the shallow end of the pool.

Today was a hot day. I was visiting Ruth and Louis [friends], whose pool invited us to cool off. Ruth and Louis headed for the deep end, and I slid carefully into the shallow end. After a few minutes, I thought I would test my balance by swimming across the shallow end of the pool. As I started to swim, I knew I was in trouble: my legs went up, and I lay facedown in the water, unable to get my head up or call for help. I blacked out. When I came to, Ruth and Louis were pulling me from the pool. I was terrified at the close call. From now on, I'll have to follow one more rule: In the water, stay close to someone who will watch for any sign of trouble.

October 1988—Today is a beautiful day, as we travel through the West. It's one of those days to be recalled often, to bring peace and calm to the soul. Whenever I'm in an especially stressful situation, I try to recall a happy experience and relive it in my mind. Often I've used the memory of a picnic on the Maine coast with Susan and Keith to calm myself. I picture how we stood in the ocean waters and let the waves come to us. We were like children, laughing, falling, and feeling the sand shift under our feet.

I remember the CAT scan I underwent when I was first diagnosed for Parkinson's, and the claustrophobia I felt as my upper body was rolled into the center of the machine. Tension and stress began to build until I closed my eyes and relived the joyful picnic by the ocean. Then I could relax. (A few years later I told Susan about my use of that memory to clear my mind of stress. She looked surprised. She, too, had used the memory of that picnic—to help her through labor during Bethany's birth.)

October 1988—Yesterday, Blaine and I visited Yellowstone National Park, and its geyser, which is so much like a centerpiece surrounded by wonders. We were thrilled to watch the geyser erupt!

At a campground in Cody, Wyoming, we spent the night, waking up today to find a crisp, sunny morning and the Grand Tetons looming outside the windows of our Winnebago. In the absence of foothills, they appeared so spectacular and so near!

After breakfast we set off on today's journey, enjoying the view of the Tetons until we came to a turnoff by a lake. Here we stopped and walked down to the edge of the water. In the absolute quiet, with the white-capped Tetons mirrored in the still, clear water, we stood for a long time, knowing that we needed to be on our way.

When we left the Tetons, the lake, and the magic to those who would journey down the road after us, we took with us the moments we spent there. They will be with us forever, ready to be recalled at a moment's notice.

May 1989—Dr. Feldman decided that it wasn't wise to put me on any more Sinemet; he started me on Permax. This was quite an experience, because I have low blood pressure and the Permax made it drop even lower, to the point that I was passing out. Then Dr. Feldman introduced Florinef to help stabilize my blood pressure.

July 1991—Blaine had become president of the Maine State Chapter of the American Parkinson Disease Association, so we attended our first national meeting of chapter presidents and coordinators in New Orleans.

September 1992—Edmonton, Alberta, Canada. Since the first edition of this book was published, Blaine and I have been invited to speak to numerous groups. We are in Edmonton to speak to the Canadian National Parkinson Convention.

November 1993—Blaine has a minor heart attack. This changes our thinking and attitude in a hurry.

September 1994—I am experiencing some "freezing" problems, and now I have to make the big decision that I didn't want to make. "Freezing" feet and gas pedals don't go well together, so it's time to give up driving.

October 1994—Blaine has a major heart attack. Now the Parkinson's patient becomes the caregiver. After angioplasty surgery, medication, a medically approved diet, and exercise, Blaine is doing much better.

June 1995—I'm having problems getting out of my swivel, rocking easy chair, so we decide that it's time to buy an electric-lift easy chair. I use the lift only when I have problems.

October 1996—Our old water bed is feeling its age, and I want something firmer, so we buy a new innerspring mattress. Blaine builds a ramp and a grab-bar on my side of the bed. This makes it easier for me to get into and out of bed, since the new mattress is several inches higher off the floor than the water bed was.

Winter 1997—Even with changes in my Parkinson's, I'm trying to live a full life. For example, we're working on this revision while in a campground in Florida.

May 1997—Because of Parkinson's, we have a new friend, an English lady who spends six months in Maine each year and the other six months back home in England. Her mother had Parkinson's, so she has been involved in English Parkinson's organizations. She gave us a lot of interesting materials relating to Parkinson's.

1998—I'm having more blood pressure problems that we haven't got under control, so I sometimes pass out without warning. I now use the wheelchair when shopping and going out.

1998—I just received a letter from Mary Baker, the president of the European Parkinson Disease Association. We had met her in Boston, and the association wants to display and advertise my book in the EPDA magazine and possibly on its Web page.

Author's note: Glenna passed away on November 25, 1998.

CHAPTER 13

With a Little Help from My Family and Friends

A faithful friend is the medicine of life.

—Ecclesiastes 6:16

I am always aware that my many relatives and friends are an important part of my life. In this chapter, I want to encourage you to pursue an active social life, not only by maintaining the relationships you have developed over the years, but by continuing to forge new relationships—with relatives with whom you have lost contact and with aquaintances you meet who share your interests.

Many people with Parkinson's retire from a busy career only to discover that their need to interact with others, which had previously been satisfied by their spouses, children, and coworkers, is now met by only a few close family members. In some cases, the spouse, too, has passed away; in others, the children live at some distance. The person with Parkinson's retreats into isolation and depression. Unhappiness is intensified when one or two individuals alone bear the entire responsibility of meeting the social and emotional needs of the person with Parkinson's and that responsibility becomes too much for them.

The very first step that you should take in forging new relationships is to join a Parkinson's support group, where you will meet other people with Parkinson's and their caregivers, who are working through problems and adjustments very similar to your own. (More about this important step in the next chapter, which is devoted to support groups.)

The next step in the search for meaningful friendships is to reach out to parents, children, brothers, sisters, cousins, nieces, and nephews—including those you haven't seen in some time. Even if your family has been torn apart by grudges or misunderstandings, don't be afraid to make the first move. Any effort you can make toward building bridges will be well spent. Sure, your family members have faults, but so does everyone. Love and accept your family members as they are, and you will enjoy their love and acceptance. Regardless of how small or large, your family and your spouse's family are important parts of your emotional support network.

Blaine, of course, is my best friend. And I am very close to my children and grandchildren. But my sisters, Doris and Donna, and my sister-in-law, Linda, are also very special friends. Whether we sisters are giggling like children, shopping the sales, just quietly talking, or even having an argument, we know that we can turn to one another with our serious problems. The first real tragedy that we shared was the death of Donna's fifteen-month-old child when she was struck by a car. We learned then the value of family support.

When I told my family that I had Parkinson's, I knew they would be supportive. Although they live at some distance, they have been very helpful, even coming down to help me with housecleaning. The thing that helps most is their devotion. They never fail to invite me to join them in activities or outings at appropriate times. When I move slowly (which is often), they are patient.

My only brother, George, was the brother everyone ought to have had. He made the most of life and was an example for all who knew him. He, too, spent a great deal of time with us. Whenever he and his wife, Linda, came to Bangor, they appeared on our doorstep, asking us to eat out with them. Whenever we go to those same restaurants now, we can't help remembering our meals and the good times with George and Linda. A few years ago, George was killed in a canoeing accident. His death has left a great void in my life, as did my father's death earlier, but I still feel Dad's and George's love for me as I call on the memory of their wisdom, humor, and words of comfort.

I'm happy to say that some of my best friends are my nieces and nephew. My nephew is Doris's eldest child. A special bond with him was formed when I lived with Doris and her family (while Blaine was away in the service), and I spent a great deal of time with my infant nephew. Recently, I wrote a letter to him explaining the bond I felt, which he understood and said that he felt, too. The letter helped to reaffirm the bond.

I developed special friendships with Donna's children as well. When they were young, Donna brought them to visit for four or five days at a time, and we enjoyed many things together, especially crafts, picnics, excursions, and games. One of our favorite activities was our annual gift exchange before Christmas. We couldn't afford expensive gifts in those days, but I made and assembled very decorative gift boxes, which my nieces looked forward to every year. They can't remember the gifts now, but they still remember the boxes. All of Donna's girls became interested in crafts, an interest they attribute to those early craft sessions, and they now come down to visit with their own children.

When you are reestablishing old ties, remember that relationships take time to develop. They are the culmination of time and effort and many shared experiences. For example, when my sisters and I went off to school and later married, we couldn't afford many long-distance telephone calls, but we wrote long letters to keep one another up-to-date on our lives, and we visited often. Even long, well-established relationships need care and attention. Maintain your correspondence with your relatives, telephone them, visit and invite them to visit you, go on excursions and eat out together, celebrate birthdays and holidays together. Be interested in their activities and successes, and be supportive in their times of trouble or discouragement. Don't be overly demanding of their time. Don't criticize or try to change them. Overlook their faults.

In addition to relatives, you need to include many friends in your support network. Friends are the people with whom you choose to share parts of your life.

Friends entered our lives in many different ways. There were the neighbors, Dana and Mary, and Marge and Ervin, whose lives meshed with ours when our children became so close that it was hard to tell which were theirs and which were ours. Eventually, they moved away, but we still get together. Whenever we need to get away, we drive down to New Hampshire or Connecticut to spend a weekend with one couple or the other. When we get together, it's as if we have never been apart. Another friend in the early group of neighbors was Florence. What would I do without Florence? Every few days she calls to say that she is going out, and I am welcome to come along. Maybe we will go out for lunch. She is the kind of friend who will rearrange her schedule, if she can, to help me.

Some friends entered my life through my career. Vivian, Ruth, Lynne, Donna, Pat C., and Pat T. are linked to my teaching. Different friends fill different needs.

We found new friends in our church in Hampden and others through Blaine's work, even before he started teaching.

Be very deliberate about keeping in touch with your old friends, and make time to see them each week or as often as possible. At the same time, establish new contacts and make new friends through church activities, interest clubs, fraternal clubs, adult education classes, and volunteer work. You need to be stimulated by other people, to interact in meaningful ways with other people, to reach out and socialize with others. What you don't want or need is a life of sitting at home alone.

As with families, relationships with friends do not just happen. Time and effort are needed. We must set aside time to see our friends, and we need to make an effort to arrange ways we can get together, whether visiting at home, meeting at a picnic or a restaurant, swimming at the Y, or going to a sports event. There are many inexpensive ways to socialize such as attending a local high school or college drama or a musical production; meeting at home for a game of Scrabble, checkers, or cards; taking a walk or a drive; or bringing a bag lunch to the park. Don't wait to be invited. Take the initiative. Do the inviting!

And, as with relatives, we must remember not to lean too heavily on any one individual; no one friend can meet all of our needs. When we have many friends, different individuals can satisfy different needs. One friend may enjoy sharing an hour or two doing crafts. One may enjoy walking. Another may like to go out for coffee and dessert. If a friend turns you down when you invite him or her to other kinds of activities, don't feel hurt or rejected. Each of us spends only the time we can comfortably spend; each of us pursues only the activities we care to pursue. Why should we expect our friends to be different?

Overlook the imperfections you discover in your friends. Make allowances for differences. We are all different, and none of us is perfect.

Remember also that friendship is a two-way street. As people with Parkinson's, we sometimes get into the rut of letting others do many things for us, and we forget what we can do for others. The truth is that we have as much to offer others as they have to offer us. Each of us has special skills and abilities acquired in our jobs and our hobbies that can be helpful to our relatives and friends. In addition, we can remember our friends' special days with little gifts, balloons, or humorous poems. When friends are ill, we can bring (or send) cards, flowers, or chicken soup. We can be caring listeners when our friends have problems. Although we can occasionally use their shoulders to cry on, we should generally avoid dwelling on gloomy thoughts when we are with them.

*   *   *

After my diagnosis in 1981, I realized that I couldn't control the fact that I had Parkinson's disease, but I could control the amount of time I might waste sitting around and wishing I didn't have it. I'm passing this thought on to you: let your Parkinson's make you a *better* person, not a *bitter* person. Seek out others who need your help. Use your time and energy to cultivate friendship. Be a friend to many people. In return, you will be surrounded by love, friendship, and emotional support.

CHAPTER 14

Support Groups: Where You Learn What Your Doctor Hasn't Time to Tell You!

People must help one another; it is nature's law.
— *Jean de La Fontaine*, Fables, *L'Âne et le Chein*

It's Sunday afternoon in the all-purpose room of a local church. A small group of about twenty people are milling about, drinking coffee and socializing. Soon they seat themselves in a circle, and the meeting begins. After new visitors are introduced and a few minutes are devoted to business, the group begins a period of sharing. This is a time when individuals have an opportunity to share with the rest of the group the successes they have experienced during the past month and to ask questions about problems to which others may have answers.

When everyone who wishes to speak has done so, the group turns its attention to the program. The program may feature a speaker who addresses a topic of importance to the members and then opens the topic to discussion and questions. Or it may be a videotaped presentation, followed by a discussion of the taped subject. Or the program may be the posing of several questions by the chairman, each question followed by a general discussion. Partway through the program, the group takes a break to move about and enjoy a cup of coffee, and after the program, there may be more socializing.

This is the monthly meeting of the Greater Bangor Parkinson's Support Group. The group is made up of people with Parkinson's and their spouses or other caregivers. A few visitors may also be present: perhaps another family member or a friend of one of the "regulars," or a new person with Parkinson's or a spouse who is coming to see what we have to offer. If a focused discussion is planned (rather than a speaker or a videotaped presentation), the group may remain as one group, or it may split up into two groups so that spouses and other caregivers can discuss their concerns separately from the people with Parkinson's. If a prominent speaker or a panel is scheduled for the program, members of other Maine support groups may have joined us for the meeting.

What is a Parkinson's support group? And how does it function? It is a group ranging in size from a dozen people to more than a hundred, who generally meet once a month to learn about the care and the treatment of Parkinson's, exchange insights and newly learned coping techniques, and offer friendship, support, and understanding to one another.

Each group is different. Some groups meet more often than once a month. Some groups follow a format similar to ours; others include ballroom dancing in their social time; some break for an exercise period; some serve baked goods, other snacks, and soft drinks, in addition to coffee. Some groups organize theater trips and outings in addition to their regular meetings. Some groups split up for general discussion: people with Parkinson's in one group and caregivers in another. Some include anyone with Parkinson's, while others limit their membership to either older patients or younger patients and their families. Some groups are for caregivers only.

Our group is small and very informal. Blaine and I cochair the meetings; we arrange for a speaker, a videotape, or a discussion. A secretary publicizes the meetings and keeps a very brief record of each meeting and a list of the names and addresses of new visitors. A treasurer handles the money. We have no dues or fees, but we set a bowl on the table for voluntary donations. One couple is kind enough to donate—and prepare—the coffee for each meeting. When members of the community pass away, mourners sometimes send donations to our group in lieu of flowers to the family. We use the money for mailing notices and to advertise our meetings. We also bought a television and a VCR for the church where we meet, with the understanding that we can use them at our meetings. We donate money for research to national Parkinson's organizations.

Our support group has given us the opportunity to learn a great deal about Parkinson's disease and what we can do for ourselves in treating it. Our speakers have included doctors, psychologists, physical therapists, occupational therapists, a hearing specialist, and a nutritionist, all speaking on various aspects of the management of Parkinson's disease. A speaker from Sandoz (a pharmaceutical company) talked to us and answered our questions about Parlodel (bromocriptine), one of its products. A representative from the Eastern Agency on Aging informed us about community services (such as adult day care) that are available to local senior citizens. A program we later held was a presentation of the care of the patient's teeth, gums, and mouth, to address the difficulty that people with Parkinson's have (because of dry mouth) in maintaining good oral hygiene.

We aren't the only learners at these programs. The speakers say that they learn a great deal from us during the discussion period when we contribute our ideas and voice our concerns.

The videotapes we rent from Parkinson's organizations have been instructive to our group. They have featured exercise programs for people with Parkinson's, roundtable discussions on Parkinson's, and doctors lecturing on Parkinson's. Some have had motivational value as well.

Our group especially looks forward to discussions and sharing. What we learn from one another is as valuable as what we learn from speakers and tapes. Everyone is anxious to share. What I value most of all is hearing others express the same things I have experienced but have not been able to communicate to people who don't have Parkinson's. No one else understands us as well as other people with Parkinson's, not even our spouses or closest family members. The sharing that we do leaves a good feeling afterward. Of course, the spouses and other caregivers feel the same way about sharing their feelings and insights. No one understands as well as others in the same role do. At the support group, even in the midst of our frustrations, we find joy and laughter, hope and determination.

In addition to our regular meetings, our members look forward to two special occasions together: the annual picnic in July and the restaurant outing during the Christmas season.

An important aspect of the support group for me is my job as cochair. It is rewarding because of the opportunities it gives me to help others in the group and to find new topics for the group to share. And as the contact person for the group, I enjoy talking to new people who have heard about the group, who call to find out more or talk about their own situations. One woman calls anonymously every few months because her husband has Parkinson's and doesn't want anyone to know. For her, calling is the next best thing to attending a support group. Someday I hope to meet her and her husband as well.

Although our group has reached many people with Parkinson's over the years, we know there are many others who choose to stay home. I think that some people are uncertain about how a support group functions. Others fear that they will become depressed by seeing people in more advanced stages of Parkinson's. If you are afraid of this, I can assure you that the support group members I've met across the country have not been depressed by others at their group meetings. Those with Parkinson's who make the effort to attend are not likely to be depressing; rather, they are usually friendly and positive. They are good role models. Most important, the support group meeting is the one place where you will find others who truly know what you and your spouse are experiencing. The good comradeship and warm feelings that are generated in support groups will allay your fears about attending.

Some years ago, my daughter, Susan, attended a meeting of our group, despite her apprehensions about what she might find there. In an observation paper that she prepared for one of her college classes, she wrote,

> I must admit I went with preconceived notions and fears: the fear of seeing and having to face in others what the progression of Parkinson's may do one day to my mother. I expected to see a group of crippled, elderly people, all shaking uncontrollably, with faces reflecting sadness and despair. I was pleasantly surprised. Parkinsonians, spouses, other family members, and friends of various ages from early fifties to mid-eighties, were present; and although various stages of Parkinson's, from undetectable to obvious, were represented, there was no sadness or despair. Yes, I know that there are many parkinsonians, especially those who have little support from family and friends, who do feel despair and resentment. But this group of individuals is trying to cope with and control this condition. They are doing it with knowledge and positive attitude, the basis of the support group. . . .
>
> The individuals in the group seem genuinely interested in learning about coping with Parkinson's, and about how each one is dealing with it. They have developed a caring attitude toward each other, and they gain strength from each other.

If you don't already belong to a support group, you are probably interested in locating or even starting one. To find the group nearest you, call or write to the national organizations with which many Parkinson's support groups are affiliated: Parkinson's Support Groups of America (PSGA), American Parkinson Disease Association (APDA), Parkinson's Educational Program (PEP), and United Parkinson Foundation (UPF). The addresses and the telephone numbers are listed in appendix A, in the back of this book.

Not all support groups are affiliated with national organizations. Check the yellow pages and the white pages of your telephone book for the "Parkinson's Support Group of [your locality]." Call neurologists in your area or the neurology department of your nearest hospital or medical center, in the hope that someone in those offices may know of an existing support group. Your own doctor may know of one.

There are hundreds of Parkinson's support groups in the United States (and many in other countries, as well). But if no support group exists in your general area, or if there is a very large one, you might like to start a new one. Today a great deal of information is available that details, in step-by-step fashion, how to start a new support group.

In early 1982, when Blaine and I first thought about starting a Parkinson's support group in the Bangor area, little printed information was available and no established group was close enough to look in on or contact for advice. Actually, we had mixed feelings about starting something we were so unfamiliar with.

In our search for information, we learned about the national organization PSGA and about its annual convention, which was to take place that year at Camp Maria on Chesapeake Bay (Maryland). At the convention, we knew we'd be able to talk to people who were familiar with support groups and how to get them started; we would also be able to determine how people felt about support groups and whether the effort would be worth our while. After some hesitation, we decided to attend the convention, and when the day came to leave for Maryland, we headed down the road, still uncertain of our feelings. As we drove closer and closer, we looked at each other and asked what we were getting into.

But we didn't turn back, and we were glad we didn't. Camp Maria was beautiful, and the people we met there were friendly, helpful, and encouraging. The advice and information we got from those around us and the feeling of closeness that we experienced during the sing-along on the last evening convinced us that a support group could be truly beneficial. Attending the convention had not been a prerequisite to starting a group, but at that time it was a good place to learn—and to get a shot of confidence.

Another source of help that we found in those early days came from Parkinson's Educational Program (PEP), founded by Charlotte Jayne Drake. PEP offered help in starting support groups and made information about Parkinson's and Parkinson's support groups available (pamphlets, newsletters, and audio and visual tapes) free of charge. Through the mail, PEP also sold books about Parkinson's, satin sheets, and other items that are useful to people with Parkinson's.

Soon, we began to act on the advice we received and laid some groundwork for a support group by gaining the help of another couple, the Watsons, who were interested in joining us and by finding a place for our first meeting in a church. In the fall of 1982, we put an announcement in the newspaper, which expressed our desire to meet with anyone interested in Parkinson's and gave the date, the time, and the place of the meeting, along with our telephone number. Several people arrived at that first meeting, all of whom, happily, are still with us.

Encouraged by a good beginning, we set a date for the next meeting, which we held at a motel. Unfortunately, this facility charged a fee that we felt we could not afford, so our third meeting was held in another church, the meeting place we have used ever since. We meet once a month on Sunday afternoons; Sunday is generally a convenient day, and the afternoon is best for us because some of our members have a long drive and don't like to travel home late at night. In the more than twenty years since we started meeting, our group has grown to about twenty regular members and a number of others who drop in from time to time. It's a cozy, informal group.

For years, our Parkinson's support group has been affiliated with both PSGA and PEP. (A group can be affiliated with several national organizations.) We also support APDA, the largest of the national groups. Affiliation with national organizations makes a group eligible for newsletters, information packets, and tape rentals, as well as other assistance. National organizations will also help groups arrange for speakers, panel discussions, and small symposia. (For example, the Maine groups were aided in holding a symposium with a panel of four Parkinson's specialists. What a wealth of information we shared that day!) APDA is unique, in that it also sends representatives to help set up a group and gives the group $300 toward its early ground-laying expenses: publicity, postage, paper supplies, refreshments, and so forth. Affiliation does not affect the way a group operates. Each group retains its autonomy and its own way of doing things.

Today if you are interested in starting a support group, you have the national organizations, other support groups, and many printed materials to help you. The first step is to contact APDA, PSGA, and PEP to tell them of your interest and ask for their free printed guides. The guide "How to Start a Parkinson's Disease Community Support Group," offered by APDA headquarters in New York, for example, is an invaluable aid. Also, you can contact another support group in a nearby area and drop in to observe the way the group operates and to talk to people. Take the telephone numbers of the officers of the club, so that you can call them later with questions.

Keep in mind that you do not have to have Parkinson's to start a support group. Many groups are started by spouses, grown children, or friends of people with Parkinson's. Some groups are started by physicians, nurses, social workers, or other professionals who are motivated to fill the need in their communities.

The next step is to find a few other people (those with Parkinson's, spouses, grown children, friends, or professionals) who are willing to help you with the tasks involved in getting started. Even one or two people may be sufficient. They can help you to contact institutions that may be able to provide a meeting place that is convenient, cost-free, and barrier-free (accessible to wheel-chairs), with adequate parking and toilet facilities. Your best bets are senior citizen centers, churches, synogogues, and Ys. You can also approach hospitals, because they have meeting rooms that can sometimes be used by groups, and you can talk to the super-intendents of apartment buildings with recreation rooms. It is also possible to hold initial meetings in a large recreation room in someone's home.

It helps if your meeting room is a cheerful place. Give each institution an idea of the day, the time, and the number of hours your group may need to use the facility, and let its representatives know that you will need to seat at least fifteen to twenty people. Determine whether the management will permit refreshments to be served and whether the facility is adequately heated in the win-ter and cooled in the summer. Keep a list of all these factors for each facility.

Once you or your helpers have obtained a meeting room and have set a date for the first meeting, you must publicize both the formation of the group and the meeting. Compose a flyer that announces the formation of a new Parkinson's support group for people with Parkinson's and their families; the date, the time, and the place of the first meeting; an invitation to all interested indi-viduals to attend; and the telephone number of the contact person (you or one of your helpers). Twenty or thirty copies of the flyer can be reproduced on someone's computer or on the photocopy machine at the library or the post office.

At least two weeks before the meeting, send copies of the flyer to local neurologists (including your own) and social service departments of local hospitals, asking them to help spread the news. Also send flyers and a short note about the purpose of your support group to the editor of the health and medicine page of the area newspaper, the local radio station, and the news depart-ment of the local TV station, all of which will probably get you some free publicity. Besides the announcement in the newspapers (which is free), you may want to pay for a short display ad to appear on the health and medicine page of the daily paper or for a classified ad in the weekly paper.

Copies of your flyer should also be pinned up on bulletin boards in post offices, libraries, churches, senior citizen centers, supermarkets, apartment complexes, pharmacies, medical centers, and other public places. Send announcements to the national organizations and to your nearest APDA Information and Referral Center; they, too, will help to publicize your group's existence.

Once you obtain a meeting room and set the date of the first meeting, you can arrange for a speaker. The speaker for the first meeting could be a chairperson or an active member of another support group, or a doctor, a nurse, or a social worker who has observed or assisted in the formation of another support group. One of the national organizations may be able to suggest a speaker or even arrange for one for your group. If you cannot obtain a speaker, you may want to use a videotaped presentation on the nature of Parkinson's support groups. You can borrow one from one of the national organizations. At the first meeting, you will probably want to limit the speaker (or the tape) to about thirty minutes and the follow-up discussion period to another thirty minutes, because so many other things will be happening. At later meetings, the speaker can be asked to give a somewhat longer presentation.

Plan for a few refreshments for the first meeting, such as coffee or punch and perhaps cake or cookies. (Can one of your helpers bake?) You will also need paper goods and plastic silverware. Someone must come to the meeting room a bit earlier than the others to set up the refreshment table and set out the packets of information provided by the national organizations you contacted. Updated flyers for the next meeting should be available, too, so that people can take them to their neighborhoods and put them up. Before people arrive, arrange the seats around a large table or in a circle. If the group becomes too large for this arrangement, use a more standard arrangement of rows the next time.

Be organized at that first meeting. Plan everything in advance.

You or your helper can greet people as they come in; get their names, addresses, and telephone numbers for your first mailing list; and direct them to the information packets and the pamphlets. If you provide peel-off name tags, people will get to know one another quickly.

As soon as you and your helpers have welcomed the guests and introduced yourselves, you should ask the guests to introduce themselves and perhaps tell everyone where they live and how long they or their family members have had Parkinson's. Then a few words can be said to establish the purposes of the support group; these are to educate members about Parkinson's disease; to maximize the quality of the lives of people with Parkinson's and their caregivers; to discover all the resources in the community that are useful to people with Parkinson's; and to enable every member to receive support and understanding.

After a brief description of the types of programs that often take place in a support group meeting, a short discussion should permit the guests to express what they would most look forward to in a support group and what kinds of programs and activities they would prefer. It would be helpful if a knowledgeable member of another support group or a volunteer from one of the national organizations were present to answer questions about the programs and the activities of support groups. But if that is not possible, use what you have learned in this chapter and in materials from national organizations, and you will be able to wing it. Every group is different, anyway.

You may want to break for refreshments at this point, or you might wait until you have heard the speaker or seen the tape. Generally, groups take a refreshment break after the speaker or the tape and then come back to their seats for the follow-up discussion and the question period. At the first meeting, however, the preliminaries may take up more time, and the break should be adjusted accordingly. Try to remember to take a short break at every meeting. Some people with Parkinson's become quite uncomfortable after sitting for extended lengths of time, and they need to move around.

Introduce your speaker (or tape), and inform the guests that there will be a discussion and a question period after the presentation. If the speaker seems to handle the discussion period well, allow him or her to handle it alone. If the speaker seems to need some help, then you or your helper should assist.

Before people leave, remind them of the date of the next meeting and ask each guest to put a flyer or two on bulletin boards in his or her neighborhood.

Preparation for the second meeting will be much easier, and for the third even more so. By then, you may want to ask for volunteers to do some of the preparatory tasks. And you may want to hold an election for officers. You have launched your Parkinson's support group!

In addition to attending support group meetings, I urge you to attend at least some of the conventions, the conferences, and the symposia organized by various organizations for people with Parkinson's and their families. The people whom you meet, the speakers, and the relaxed atmosphere at these gatherings all contribute to an uplifting experience.

Besides the PSGA Annual Convention that Blaine and I attended in 1982, we have gone to two more. In the mid-1980s, we attended our second convention, this time in Blowing Rock, North Carolina. We had no mixed feelings as we drove to that convention, but we did feel uneasy about the narrow roads without guard rails that wound around the mountains. When we arrived safely at our destination and went to register, it was so nice to hear people say, "I know you! You were here before! You're from Maine!" At the convention, we acquired a great deal of new information and new enthusiasm to share with our local group, and we had a delightful vacation, too.

More recently, we attended our third convention in Yucaipa, California, during a vacation trip in our Winnebago. It was our first visit to California. When we arrived at the convention site, we felt as if we were at a reunion. We renewed old friendships and also made new ones, such as with a couple from Los Angeles. These new friends invited us to their home and their local support group meeting.

The atmosphere of this convention, like that of the others, was relaxed and serene. The pace was slow, the rest periods adequate. At the same time, the convention was very productive, with excellent sessions and opportunities to chat with the speakers during breaks.

Among the speakers was one from the National Institutes of Health, who spoke about the latest Parkinson's research and who was asked by the group to extend his talk into the evening. He agreed, saying that he felt it was important to spend time with the people for whom he is conducting research.

Other speakers included two people with Parkinson's who had undergone adrenal tissue brain implants and talked about their experiences. They maintained that although they were not cured, they now had a sense of well-being that they had not experienced before the operation. Both said that they would do it over again. Their wives also spoke. When we headed east again, we had a great deal to share with our local support group, and we looked forward to it!

CHAPTER 15

Is There Life with Parkinson's?

Let us then be up and doing
  With a heart for any fate;
Still achieving, still pursuing,
  Learn to labor and to wait.

—Henry Wadsworth Longfellow, Psalm of Life

Is there life with Parkinson's disease? I'm writing this book to assure you that you can enjoy a productive and fulfilling life! There are so many reasons you must decide to live effectively and commit yourself to building into life the quality that you desire.

The outlook for people with Parkinson's is better today than it has ever been before. Just thirty-five years ago, the prospects were bleak. The medications available then were not much help, and research lagged. With the arrival of Sinemet, the quality of life was vastly improved. In spite of the side effects of overmedication for some, Sinemet permitted most Parkinson's patients to go on with their lives and permitted doctors to offer hope when they announced, "You have Parkinson's."

Today, Sinemet has help from bromocriptine (Parlodel) and pergolide (Permax), which enable people with Parkinson's to take less Sinemet and to enjoy its effectiveness longer, without as many side effects as before. Combination drug therapy also helps to reduce the "off" periods. In addition, the drug deprenyl may postpone the need to start taking Sinemet and helps people who are already taking Sinemet. The drug holiday provides relief from overmedication. One of the most exciting breakthroughs was when scientists perfected methods of implanting dopamine-producing fetal neurons into the brain of a person with Parkinson's. In 2003, a study of a surgical procedure known as deep-brain stimulation reported that the procedure's benefits—reduced tremor, improvement in rigidity, and less need for medication—last five years in many patients. And soon we may even see substances produced by genetically engineered cells repairing damaged nerve tissue and helping to reverse the course of Parkinson's. The prospects are really good!

Still, the immediate outlook for individuals differs. The number and the severity of symptoms, the pattern of the disease, and the speed of progression differ for each person. Nevertheless, there is a life with quality, if the individual with Parkinson's resolves to make it so.

As someone with Parkinson's today, I don't feel that the quality of my life is less than it was before I had Parkinson's. It's just different. I've had to adapt and find new avenues. I've had to get around the problem of bouts of low energy and accept the fact that I can't do everything I used to do. Yet I can often do more than I think I can.

I'm reminded of a recent visit to a friend and her two-year-old daughter. Every time my friend asked her tot to do something, the child replied, "Can't do!" How many times do we people with Parkinson's say, "Can't do," and then go on to prove that we can? I can "do," but I do things differently than I once did.

For example, I've had to modify the amount of entertaining I do. As a people-oriented person, I used to have many visitors in our home. The number was never too many. When the children were small, I made muffins and coffee at midmorning and invited the whole neighborhood to stop by. I enjoyed that, and I'm glad I had the energy to do it. Today, I still enjoy midmorning coffee, but I invite only one or two of my friends on any one morning, and I skip the baking. Who needs the calories, anyway?

We used to have many temporary guests (student teachers, foreign students, and visiting relatives) living with us for various lengths of time. Our students from Hampden Academy came for cookouts and other gatherings. Friends and family came for dinner. We still have occasional overnight guests (who are welcome to prepare their own breakfasts from supplies I have on hand). And we still have friends or family members over for dinner, but we choose easy menus, such as casseroles and salads, much of which we prepare ahead of time, or we have an "everybody help" meal, for which each guest is happy to bring a dish. The food is incidental; we come together to enjoy one another's company.

Another activity I love is shopping—a love that dates back to my childhood when I stood in front of Harry Hart's General Store on Saturday nights, trying to decide how to spend my pennies. As an adolescent, I remember the hours my sister and I studied the Sears Roebuck catalog before spending the money we had earned picking potatoes. Later, I became an expert at zipping around the stores, covering all bases, in order to catch the great buys. Sometimes I went with Susan; we really loved our shopping trips, especially when we had time for lunch together, laughing when we had spent our allotted money down to the last cent. Today, I think the cartoon showing the shopper confronting "so many stores, so little time!" was made for me. I'm not about to give up shopping because of Parkinson's. It's still a special part of my life, but I do it differently. I take shorter trips and more frequent rests. The people I go with understand my limitations. They know my walk might become a slow shuffle at any time. They know I need to break up the time by having coffee or lunch or by just sitting a while and "people watching." I do a little preplanning.

And I avoid trying on clothes in the store (if they don't fit, they can be returned). Recently, I tried on one outfit while Blaine waited patiently outside the dressing room. When I finally emerged from the dressing room, he admitted, "I'm glad you didn't try on two." But just in case I do decide to try things on, I go shopping in clothes that are easy to get off and on. Susan and I still laugh when we find enough super buys to use up every allotted dollar.

The biggest adaptation I made to maintain the quality of my life was to retire from teaching. I had loved teaching, especially during my last years at Hampden Academy. I brought experience, maturity, and confidence to that position and felt good about my accomplishments, but the regimen of teaching while coping with Parkinson's had become too stressful. I became convinced that I could lead a more fulfilling life if I retired. So I said good-bye to a wonderful part of my life and looked forward to other wonderful things ahead. Immediately, there were trade-offs. I gave up teaching, but I also gave up rushing off to work each morning. What luxury to stay in bed and read the newspaper! I even did the cross-word puzzle. Blaine brought me my morning coffee. I reached for the TV's remote control and flicked on the morning news. I felt pampered. During the day, I worked on projects and activities that I'd had little time for during my teaching years. And I spent more time with my grandchildren and my ailing mother. Eventually, I also gave more time to other people with Parkinson's and their spouses who, over the years, have called to talk earnestly about their problems.

My friends often ask whether I miss teaching. Yes, I do miss the students and the staff with whom I worked. But the home economics teachers have made it comfortable for me to drop by any time. They invite my input in the planning of new courses. They invite me to family suppers, parties, and after-school coffees. Sometimes I attend area home economics meetings. Thus, I do not feel isolated from my colleagues or my professional interests. I have good memories of the past, but I live in the present; I enjoy today.

Observing other people with Parkinson's, I believe that because of early conditioning and the threat to the ego, men have a harder time deciding to retire and apply for disability than women do. Fortunately, new medications enable people with Parkinson's to continue working longer than before. When full-time work becomes too difficult, part-time work can be considered. Some people may want to look for employment that offers a very flexible schedule. Some may want to develop a business at home that permits them to work at their own pace. Still others may want to stay home and help run the household. The fully retired person who has Parkinson's will want to find other outlets through which to build a productive life: part-time volunteer work (with a flexible schedule); active membership in a club, a church group, or a civic organization; social activities; gardening; a hobby or a craft; travel; or family activities.

Studies show that strong family and social ties, along with meaningful volunteer work for others, promotes health and well-being. The retired person with Parkinson's may wish to devote some time each week to a community organization or a hospital or to an individual who needs help, such as a homebound or blind person, a child who needs tutoring, or an illiterate adult who is trying to learn to read (Literacy Volunteers). Social service agencies can help to locate such individuals if none are known in the neighborhood. The retiree may wish to read to a child or an adult in the noncontagious ward of a hospital or become an "adoptive grandparent" to a child in an orphanage or a children's shelter. There are many ways to help isolated or handicapped people.

In Brooklyn, New York, there was a woman named Dora Moskowitz (who didn't have Parkinson's), who had helped homebound neighbors in a large apartment building for more than forty years. She had shopped and cooked meals for them, mailed their letters, delivered rent checks, and helped them in many ways to stay at home, rather than in institutions. As a result, she was probably the youngest, ablest eighty-four-year-old in Brooklyn. People with Parkinson's may not be able to do as much as Dora did but helping others in whatever ways we can keeps us active, involved, and healthy. It contributes to a positive attitude and gives us a sense of purpose.

I have found many avenues to a productive life since I retired. One opportunity came when two young friends started a preschool in Hampden and asked for my advice in setting it up and developing the curriculum. I enjoyed being a "consultant." Now and then, I drop in to help, and I proudly wear the Highland Preschool sweatshirt with the teddy bear on it (to the delight of my grandchildren, who are graduates of the school).

I serve on the board of directors of the Good Samaritan Agency in Bangor, which is involved in placing children for adoption, as well as helping single parents. I have also served on planning committees of various community organizations, such as the March of Dimes, Family Planning, and high school conferences dealing with teen problems. Once I helped to plan a conference titled "Menopause and Beyond" for a women's center. I have spoken to associations (such as the Junior League of Women and other women's groups) on family life, teaching, and other areas that interest me. I also serve on committees at our church.

Before my son-in-law, Keith, joined Atwood Builders, I did the bookkeeping and the paperwork for the family business. Bookkeeping is not my strong suit, so I was glad to give that up.

Two awards that I won have helped to keep me thinking positively. In 1982, early in my Parkinson's, I received the Distinguished Service Award at Hampden Academy (the high school at which I taught). I was thrilled to receive the award but worried that my Parkinson's would interfere with future service. Nevertheless, seven years later I was named Woman of the Year by the Beta Sigma Phi sorority. This award was very meaningful to me, for it confirmed that I had not let Parkinson's stop me.

I was sponsored for Beta Sigma Phi's award by my friend Lynne Carlisle, whose eighteen-year-old daughter is no stranger to handicaps. (She has cerebral palsy but, through parental love and care, has reached levels of accomplishment that truly surprise her doctors.) At the annual dinner, Lynne read a paper explaining why she thought I deserved the award. I was touched most by her closing comments:

> Glenna has inspired me both as a fellow professional and as an individual. She has helped me become a better teacher and a better person. I have been impressed at the many times she has overcome adversity in her life and never given up. Her solution to being depressed or "down" is to help someone else. Even when her physical problems seem to be a burden, she always says, "There is someone whose problems are worse than mine."

I treasure Lynne's comments.

Almost any situation offers some good to those who are caught up in it. My Parkinson's made Blaine and me aware of what we were doing with our time. It made us reexamine our priorities. We looked around and saw people who for too long had put off things they really wanted to do, only to find at last that they would never do them because of some change in health or financial circumstances. We asked ourselves what we really wanted to do and decided that we wanted to travel.

Years ago, we had succumbed to the camping bug; we camped with family and friends all around the state of Maine. The next step, we decided, would be to buy a motor home to do more extensive travel around the United States. In the years since we made that decision, we have taken two long trips each year (one in the spring and one in the fall), as well as several smaller trips, seeing a different area on each trip. We have enjoyed all of the United States, except for Hawaii, and we have been to most of the Canadian provinces.

On the road, Blaine relaxes. I write for long stretches without interruption. I'm amazed at how easily I can write in the Winnebago (no telephones, no meetings to attend, no kids—although I miss them), just the hum of the motor, the beautiful landscape for inspiration, and the secure feeling of seeing Blaine at the wheel. From time to time, he reaches over and touches my hand. I read aloud what I have written, and he gives me suggestions or encouragement.

We keep our schedule very flexible when we travel. We allow time for detours to interesting places that we hear about along the road. Sometimes, we look up old friends and relatives.

Oklahoma was the destination of one of our long fall trips, so that we could visit Blaine's half sister, Thurley, whom Blaine had not seen in over forty years and whom I had never met. We had a lovely visit with Thurley, her husband, Jim, and part of her family, and they showed us the museums and the state of Oklahoma. We are grateful for the time we spent with them, as both Thurley and Jim died the following year. That was one trip we were glad we hadn't put off to a later time!

Florida, along with Disney World, is one of our favorite trips. We never tire of visiting the "magical kingdom" or sight-seeing along Florida's endless coastline with its beaches. We finish by visiting our longtime friends Toni and Basil for a few days. Of course, there are many wonderful detours between here and Florida, as well.

Our fall expeditions have always been westward. On one outstanding trip, we traced the background of Laura Ingalls Wilder, the author of the *Little House* books on which the television series *Little House on the Prairie* is based. We had never traveled beyond Florida or the Great Lakes states before. Seeing the vastness of the Great Plains and the size of the farming and ranching operations was a new experience for us. We left the interstate highway and traveled along smaller roads, where people waved at us as we passed them. When I mentioned to a couple in a Nebraska town how friendly everyone seemed to be, the response was that people have plenty of time to be friendly. On another trip we experienced the beauty of Colorado as we wound around that state's difficult mountain roads. The mile-high city of Denver has a beautiful backdrop: the Rocky Mountains. It was warm, in the upper

80s, but you could see snow-capped peaks in the distance. After we left Denver and headed for Leadville, via the Loveland Pass and the Eisenhower Tunnel, it began to snow. This turned into a blizzard, with two-foot snowbanks lining the roads. The highlight of the trip was Leadville, Colorado, a town to which my grandfather migrated in 1898. In Leadville, my grandfather worked as a teamster and married my grandmother, who had followed him to Colorado with her handmade wedding gown packed carefully in her luggage. There, too, my aunt Alta was born, but before Grammie had her next baby, the high altitude became too hard for her to take, and the family of three moved back to Maine. Parts of Leadville are the same as when my grandparents lived there. We took a tape-recorded guided tour and quickly learned that at such a high elevation, I had to take it slowly. I found my grandparents' names listed as citizens of the town in the Leadville library, learned the name of my grandfather's employer, and found the area where Gramp worked. We found the street where my grandparents had lived and the area where the mine was located. The old city directory told us when they had lived there and mentioned that my grandfather had driven a team of horses to haul timbers to shore up the mine. I also located the site of my grandparents' tar paper shack, where Grammie boarded some of the workers. I marveled that so much of our history had been recorded and preserved for so long in Leadville. We had another learning experience when we stayed in a campground in Breckenridge. Knowing the temperature would drop at night, Blaine set the thermostat and turned on the furnace. During the night, I woke up and told Blaine I was cold. I asked whether he had set the furnace. Checking it, he found that the furnace would not start, even though the gauge indicated that a little less than a quarter-tank of gas remained.

The next day Blaine had the furnace checked in Colorado Springs, but the technician found nothing wrong. When we told him where we'd spent the previous night, he said that at an elevation of 10,000 feet or higher, we hadn't had sufficient gas to make enough pressure for the furnace to work. Another lesson learned.

As you drive down those mountains, the grade may be steep for several miles. Blaine heeded the signs and geared down the motor home to avoid burning up the brakes. We had some white-knuckle driving, but the views were worth it.

We also visited the U.S. Air Force Academy in Colorado Springs and met a cadet who used to be one of Blaine's students. It was a very interesting place.

I want to reminisce here for a minute. Each time we cross this great country of ours, I always think of the pioneers and their struggle westward. Here we are, traveling with all the comforts of home—air conditioner, fully stocked refrigerator, and so on. We talked about the hardships of the pioneers and the fact that many never lived to see the fruition of their dreams.

From Colorado Springs we went south through Pueblo, Walsenburg, and the mountains again, through Wolf Creek Pass to see the great sand dunes, and then on to the cliff dwellings at Mesa Verde National Park.

The park sits high on a mesa in a canyon, with air so clear and the sky such a deep blue, you can see forever. I decided that it wasn't smart for me to climb the ladders to see inside the cliff dwellings, so we walked the trails, visited other ruins, and learned about the Native Americans. It was amazing to look up at the cliffs and wonder how they got rocks up there to build their homes.

We headed northwest to Salt Lake City, not only to see the country but to visit the genealogy library of the LDS Church. We took an interesting tour of the city and the capitol building, but the highlight was hearing the Mormon Tabernacle Choir sing. We were lucky even to get into the tabernacle, because of the crowds.

It was fascinating to learn that this massive, dome-shaped building had been built with no nails, spikes, or any metal fasteners to support the large roof.

Next, we went south to visit some of the national parks in Utah. Each park is unique, and its beauty must be experienced firsthand. Pictures never capture the feeling. As we listened to the news on the radio, we learned that a major snowstorm was coming, so we decided to visit Las Vegas. Vegas is a great place to take in some shows and eat out, and you can always play the slots.

After leaving Las Vegas, we went to see Lake Mead and Boulder Dam—what a massive structure! Especially from the vantage point of standing at the top and looking down the face of the dam to the power house and the Colorado River below.

On we drove to the Grand Canyon. When we stood at the lip of the canyon's southern rim and looked down to the great river and across to the north rim—in one place the distance is thirteen miles—we felt very small and insignificant. We stayed there two days, so we were able to see light and colors transform the canyon walls as the sun's angle changed.

At one point we sat and watched people and mules trek to the bottom of the canyon. By the time they got there, they appeared to be the size of ants.

(After we got home, one of Blaine's male coworkers, who knew that I had Parkinson's, said in an offhanded way, "Well, why didn't you [Blaine] go to the bottom of the canyon?" Blaine responded that he hadn't thought about it, because he was too happy to see the canyon and spend two days there with me.)

Then it was on to the Painted Desert and the Petrified National Park. We found it difficult to imagine that what is now a desert was once a large forest. Outside the park, Blaine bought a piece of petrified wood to put in a rock chimney that he later built at home.

By writing about our travels, I'm trying to portray some of the great times Blaine and I have had since my diagnosis. When you find out that you have a debilitating disease like Parkinson's, it isn't the end of the world. You don't have to give up. You can go places and do things and just modify your activities, if necessary.

"So, you didn't get to the bottom of the canyon." Well, no, but we did see it.

Touring San Diego with our niece Angie was memorable, as was seeing San Jose and San Francisco with our cousin Al. In-between, we enjoyed the beautiful California coast, and afterward, we wouldn't have wanted to miss following the Oregon Trail eastward.

The United States is a glorious country. And who better to share it with than Blaine? We are so fortunate!

Quite a bit of our traveling has combined our vacations with attending Parkinson's conferences and speaking to Parkinson's groups. We have spoken to groups in a dozen or more states, as well as in Canada. When we get a request to speak somewhere, Blaine figures out whether we can combine it with a vacation and see some of the country at the same time. I've received notes and letters from people who have read my book and invited us to stop and visit them. Our Christmas card list now includes new friends whom we have met all over the United States.

Not everything has been perfect, though. Once when we were visiting some friends with Parkinson's in Sacramento, the weather was very hot and humid. After leaving our friends and heading back to the campground, I decided to use the bathroom in the motor home while Blaine drove.

Because of the heat, the humidity, and my low blood pressure, I passed out. At that moment, Blaine was driving in city traffic and had no place to stop. It took a few minutes before he found a place to pull over to the curb, and by then, I had come to. He decided that in the future, whenever I needed to use the bathroom, I would do it only when he could pull over and be available if I needed him.

I want to share more of our good times on the road. We spent one night on a mountain, looking out over the lights of Las Cruces, New Mexico. It was like Christmas. We felt really small and unimportant walking among the giant redwoods and sequoias, knowing that these trees had been alive here before Christ's time on earth.

I remember the beauty and the grandeur of Yosemite National Park and the massive granite El Captain. Strolling through the Olympia rain forest. Listening to the wolves. Seeing Old Faithful and other magnificent sights and animals of Yellowstone National Park.

Or sitting by a lake, absorbing the beauty of the Grand Tetons and their reflections in the water. I had one of Blaine's slides made into a large photograph that now hangs over his dresser. It's one of the first things he sees in the morning.

One spring we were asked to speak to a Parkinson's group in Charleston, South Carolina. We took some extra time and drove down Skyline Drive and Blue Ridge Parkway. The rhododendrons and azaleas were beautiful! We met a young pre-med student whose Parkinson's had first manifested before she became a teenager, but it wasn't properly diagnosed until her first year of college. She was the second young woman I'd met who hadn't been diagnosed for several years after her symptoms began.

The biggie was our trip to Alaska. We had talked about this with our friends Ervin and Marge Lenentine for quite sometime. I was beginning to notice progression in my Parkinson's, so we decided to take the trip rather than put it off any longer.

It was during this time that Dr. Feldman found it necessary to add Permax to my medicine, causing my low blood pressure to drop even more. Before the Florinef was added to help stabilize it, I was passing out as often as five or six times a day.

I discussed this with Dr. Feldman before our trip, and he said jokingly, "Stand her on her head and she will come around in a minute."

I said, "We can stay home and I can pass out, or we can go to Alaska and maybe I'll pass out, and maybe I won't." Except for my passing out once and falling once, the trip went off without a hitch.

We left Maine and drove south to meet the Lenentines at their place in Connecticut. The next day, the two motor homes headed for Alaska. On our way across the northern part of the United States, we visited Mount Rushmore and Bear Country.

We spent our wedding anniversary in Calgary, Alberta, Canada, and the next day drove to Banff National Park and Lake Louise. From there, we went up the Icefield Highway to the Columbia Icefield, taking a special bus onto the Athabasca Glacier. Standing there on the roof of Canada, we learned that the glacier's water flowed into three different oceans: the Pacific, the Arctic, and the Atlantic.

Then we drove on to Jasper National Park, where we had to wait for mountain sheep to move out of the road, and we followed the Yellowstone Highway through the city of Prince George. Next, we headed up the John Hart Highway to the Alaskan Highway a little above Fort Saint John. The Alaskan Highway is no longer the same as it was during World War II. Most of it is now either tarred or hot-topped; what little gravel road remains is well-maintained and smooth. If you like "God's Country," you will love this area, with its lakes, rivers, waterfalls, mountains, glaciers, and wild animals.

On the way to Valdez, we stopped at the top of the pass. What a view, standing above the clouds! People were throwing snowballs from banks that lay alongside the road.

We drove through a canyon and saw several waterfalls. When we camped next to the harbor, Blaine went over to watch commercial fishing boats unloading salmon.

Later we visited one of our former students. I asked him what the usual snowfall was, and he said, "Three hundred-and-some-odd inches." Grinning, he added, "We had an unusual winter last year, with over five hundred inches of snow. We just tunneled out of our homes."

The next day, Ervin and Blaine went fishing over by the Valdez Oil Terminal and caught several good-sized salmon from the shore. This part of Alaska is much like the irregular coast of Maine, where you either take a ferry to reach the next land mass or you backtrack.

Later we took a detour through Copper Canyon. Crossing a bridge, we saw boats coming in with king salmon, so, needless to say, the men did a U-turn in a hurry. Ervin went up river that afternoon and caught a fifty-pound king salmon.

It took Blaine all afternoon to hike up the glacier-fed river. He did get up enough courage to return the next morning and caught a thirty-five-pound salmon, calling the catch "the thrill of a lifetime."

Blaine and Ervin decided to freeze our salmon and send it home by air freight so that our families could have a big salmon feast when we got home.

Anchorage was an interesting city. After traveling through rural Alaska, you come into a modern city of more than a quarter-million people. It's a pretty city with a lot of flowers and greenery. When I show people pictures of Anchorage, they can't believe how many flowers are growing that far north. But when you think of the midnight sun and the fact that Alaska gets so many hours of daylight, it's easy to see why things grow so rapidly.

We camped in Homer, with a stop in Seward, a visit to Portage Glacier, then on to Denali Park. We were lucky and were able to see the "Great One," without any clouds obscuring it. What a magnificent sight! At 20,320 feet, Mt. McKinley is the highest mountain in North America. We didn't go into Denali, because at that point, we learned that my mother had passed away.

Blaine and I decided that because our entourage included the motor home, our friends, and our dog, I would fly home alone and later fly back to meet him. When he called our daughter and son and told them to meet me at the airport, they were upset, not realizing how much I had improved physically since we started the trip.

Blaine arranged for the airline to have a wheelchair available when I changed planes. That proved to be a big bonus when I flew back to meet him in Edmonton, Alberta. He was sitting in the waiting room while I went through Customs. After a few minutes, the airplane crew emerged from Customs; then a flight attendant brought me out in a wheelchair. Passengers in wheelchairs are usually the last to leave the plane, but the attendant wheeled me to the head of the line. In a few minutes I had passed through Customs and joined Blaine.

We had wanted to stop in Edmonton to see the world's largest shopping mall. What a sight! Eight hundred stores, theaters, hotels, and restaurants, as well as an entertainment area with merry-go-rounds, a roller coaster, and other rides and things to do. And, oh, yes, the Drop of Death, a ride where you sit strapped in a cage, soar to the top, and free-fall about five stories. (A few years after this trip, we returned to Edmonton, Alberta, to speak to the Canadian National Parkinson Convention.)

We eventually came back into the United States by way of Minot, North Dakota.

Again, I want to remind you that the reason I wrote this chapter is to show you that we had some great times and you don't have to give up living just because you have Parkinson's.

I don't want to give the impression that you need a motor home to travel. Our friend Faylene travels with her sister or a friend on chartered bus trips. She finds the other passengers to be understanding and helpful. Other friends, who are members of our support group, traveled with their daughter and her family to Disney World by plane. There, in a visit they will all remember, they paced themselves so that Grandpa and four-year-old Chris wouldn't become overtired.

We, too, have traveled by plane, when we went to England to obtain medication and see London for a week. We flew at night when there were many empty seats and we could stretch out.

When you are 30,000 feet over the Atlantic Ocean, silly thoughts flit through your mind. Before I dozed off, I thought about the pills in my purse. What if we crashed and I survived? I wouldn't last long in the water without my medication. Casually, I dug the pills out of my purse and slipped them into my pocket. If we went down, my pills and I would go together!

In London, the people, the architecture, the history, the shopping, and the atmosphere were worth the trip. We were surprised at how clean the air was. We traveled on the "tube," the metropolitan underground train. We shopped at Harrod's and were awed by St. Paul's Cathedral, Westminster Abbey, and the Tower of London. Because genealogy is one of my interests, we spent some time at St. Catherine's, a registry where all the English and Scottish births, deaths, and marriages as far back as 1837 are recorded. Although we stayed at our hotel in the evenings and went to bed early, we did go out one evening to see a play at a London theater.

We had only one difficult time in London, and that was caused by my bad judgment. It was Friday, our last day, and we were shopping(!). I knew that my "on" time was about to end, but we had talked about going back to Harrod's before returning to the hotel, and I assured Blaine that I would be all right. Although it was 5:30 P.M. and dark, we took the tube to Harrod's. By the time we got into the store, I was almost collapsing. I waited in the store while Blaine tried to hail a taxi, only to learn that one can't find an unoccupied taxi in London on Friday night. A policeman finally found one for us, and we sped back to our hotel, where I immediately ran a hot bath to soak in. (Soaking in a hot bath is my longtime treatment for stiffness.) I reflected on the very real need to avoid overdoing things. With Parkinson's, you have to take extra precautions. Allow plenty of time for your activity. Recognize danger signals, such as when you begin to slow down. Practice relaxation techniques.

The trip home was also difficult. I was well rested when we arrived at the airport early Saturday afternoon, but the takeoff was delayed. We waited for three hours in the terminal and then for another hour on the plane. This time the plane was full, and Blaine and I had center seats. Squeezed between Blaine and a young woman, I found no room in which to wiggle around, but worse than that, the plane was stuffy and getting hotter and hotter.

Within an hour after takeoff, I was claustrophobic. At last, I struck up a conversation with the young lady beside me. I learned that she was a Cambridge student who studied and wrote poetry and was on her way home for Christmas vacation. Gradually, I relaxed. She was my lifesaver. When we arrived in Boston, there was another long wait while we retrieved our luggage and cleared Customs. (I share this experience with you not to deter you from traveling but to encourage you to plan ahead for the best, most comfortable time and means of travel. Christmas vacation and other holidays are *not* the best time. International air travel is more difficult in many ways than air travel within the United States. Although I didn't know it then, we people with Parkinson's are eligible for wheelchair service, which we ought to call ahead to request, because it will whiz us and our companions past lines and through Customs. We can order special dietary meals, too, when we call ahead. If you prefer to travel by train, Amtrak has removable seats that create space for a wheelchair.)

In the airport, Susan, Keith, and the grandchildren were waiting for us. A rope held back the welcoming crowd, but that didn't keep Bethany and Elissa from ducking under and rushing to greet Grandma and "Pa." We enjoyed our royal welcome!

I have talked a great deal about travel because that is the dream that we pursue. But everyone has ideas of his or her own, and I want to encourage each of you to pursue your ideas and let them enrich your life. You may look forward to pulling together the details of your family history and recording them on tape for your children or grandchildren. You may dream of buying or assembling a telescope to watch the planets and the stars. You may be waiting for the right time to build a little greenhouse to grow exotic plants or to undertake some other horticultural project. Don't wait any longer. Do it!

Even if you have no special dream, develop ideas that you can pursue. Start a Parkinson's support group in your area. Start a film club: rent videos of the best films and view them in a different member's home each week or each month; follow the viewing with a discussion and refreshments. (Any special interest club could be held in members' homes in the same way.) Compile a cookbook for your daughter or granddaughter. Take up the construction of birdhouses and birdfeeders from woodcraft kits purchased in hobby stores. Put a birdfeeder outside your window and see how many species of birds visit each season. (Make sure the feeder is hanging from a rope, rather than being stationary, so that squirrels and other animals don't take over.)

Remember the toy electric trains that can be set up to run on tracks on a big table? Remember how dads and granddads used to set them up in the basement (for the kids, or so they said!) and how they would fill the tracks with bridges, tunnels, crossing lights, stations, and wonderful gadgets? How about setting up a train system yourself? (You can always say it's for the grandchildren!) If you have no space for trains, you may be interested in radio-controlled toy cars or airplanes. These can be propelled in the backyard, the park, or even the driveway.

Do you have boxes of photographs and snapshots stored away in closets? Now is a good time to sort them, divide them into piles for each child, and put them into albums that your children and grandchildren will treasure. You may want to write captions identifying the people and the places depicted in each shot. Stories, especially humorous ones about the occasions and activities captured on the film, can be enclosed in the albums as well. (Duplicates can be made of the best snapshots.)

There are so many activities worth pursuing. Correspond with a new pen pal in another country, and learn all you can about that country. Plan to redecorate that one room in your house that you never had time to beautify before. Do a genealogical search of your family. Take an adult education course or two each year (courses of every description are offered at high schools, colleges, museums, botanical gardens, and zoos). Write to senators and congressmen about issues that you think are important. (One issue you may want to write about is the high cost of many Parkinson's medications and people's need for help in meeting this expense.)

Walk. Swim with a companion. Design clothes for people with Parkinson's and other disabilities and send the designs to large department stores or mail-order houses; suggest that they start a "special needs" line of clothing. Keep a list of upcoming cultural and social events on your refrigerator or bulletin board and on your calendar, and attend as many as you feel able to. Involve your friends and other people with Parkinson's in your activities as often as possible. If you are active and involved, your positive attitude will rub off on those around you.

You did not choose to have Parkinson's, but you can choose how to live with it. Find the right doctor, join a support group, start an exercise program, eat to live, build your family relationships and friendships, pursue the activities that have meaning to you, and you will find that, yes, there is a life with Parkinson's. Only you can decide to make it happen!

Parkinson's Self-Help Organizations in the United States

American Parkinson Disease
  Association, Inc. (APDA)
60 Bay Street, Suite 401
Staten Island, NY 10301
718-981-8001
800-223-2732
www.apdaparkinson.org

Central Ohio Parkinson Society
3166 Redding Road
Columbus, OH 43221
614-481-8829

Michigan Parkinson Foundation
3990 John Road
Detroit, MI 48201
313-745-2000

National Parkinson Foundation,
  Inc.
1501 N.W. 9th Avenue/Bob Hope
  Road
Miami, FL 33136-1494
305-547-6666
800-327-4545
www.parkinson.org
(NPF affiliate chapters are in
  Orange County, Calif.; Mt.
  Diablo, Walnut Creek, Calif.;
  Redding, Calif.; the Sacramento
  Valley, Calif.; Kansas City, Mo.;
  Topeka, Kan.; Cape Cod, Mass.;
  and Washington, D.C.)

Parkinson's Disease Foundation
  (PDF)
William Black Medical Research
  Building
710 West 168th Street
New York, NY 10032-9982
212-923-4700
800-457-6676

Parkinson's Educational Program
3501 Lake Eastbrook Boulevard
  SE, No. 144
Grand Rapids, MI 49546
616-954-8077
800-617-8711
800-344-7872 (national)

Parkinson's Support Groups of
  America (PSGA)
11376 Cherry Hill Road, #204
Beltsville, MD 20705
301-937-1545

United Parkinson Foundation and
  the International Tremor
  Foundation
833 West Washington Boulevard
Chicago, IL 60607
312-733-1893

Young Parkinson's Support
  Network of California
APDA Young Parkinson's I & R
  Center
1041 Foxenwood Drive
Santa Maria, CA 93455
800-223-9776

OTHER ORGANIZATIONS

Michael J. Fox Foundation
  for Parkinson's Research
Grand Central Station
P.O. Box 4777
New York, NY 10163
212-213-3525
www.michaeljfox.org

Parkinson's Action Network
822 College Avenue, Suite C
Santa Rosa, CA 95404
707-544-1994

Parkinson's Action Network
300 North Lee Street, Suite 500
Alexandria, VA 22314
703-518-8877
800-850-4726
www.parkinsonsaction.org

Parkinson Alliance
211 College Road East, 3rd Floor
Princeton, NJ 08540
609-688-0870
800-579-8440
www.parkinsonalliance.net

Parkinson's Institute
1170 Morse Avenue
Sunnyvale, CA 94089-1605
408-734-2800
800-786-2958
www.parkinsonsinstitute.org

Parkinson's Resource
  Organization
74-090 El Paso, Suite 102
Palm Desert, CA 92260-4135
760-773-5628

Worldwide Education &
  Awareness for Movement
  Disorders (WE MOVE)
204 West 84th Street
New York, NY 10024
212-875-8312
800-437-6682
www.wemove.org

American Parkinson Disease Association Information and Referral Centers

ALABAMA

Birmingham
APDA Information and Referral
  Center
619 19th Street S
Birmingham, AL 35249
205-934-9100
www.neuro.uab.edu

ARIZONA

Tucson
APDA Information and Referral
  Center
University of Arizona
Department of Neurology
616 N. Country Club Road,
  Suite C
Tucson, AZ 85716
520-326-5400
800-541-4960
www.azapda.org

ARKANSAS

Hot Springs
APDA Information and Referral
  Center
St. Joseph's Regional Health
  Center
210 Woodbine
Hot Springs, AR 71901
501-318-1690
800-407-9295

CALIFORNIA

Fountain Valley
APDA Information and Referral
  Center
Orange Coast Memorial Medical
  Center
9940 Talbert Avenue, Suite 204
Fountain Valley, CA 92708
877-610-2732
714-378-5061
www.pmdi.org

Laguna Hills
APDA Information and Referral
    Center
Saddleback Memorial Medical
    Center
24451 Health Center Drive
Laguna Hills, CA 92863
877-610-2732
714-378-5061
www.pmdi.org

Long Beach
APDA Information and Referral
    Center
Long Beach Memorial Medical
    Center
2801 Atlantic Avenue
Long Beach, CA 90801
877-610-2732
714-378-5061
www.pmdi.org

Los Angeles
APDA Information and Referral
    Center
Cedars-Sinai Medical Center
8631 West Third Street,
    Suite 1145E
Los Angeles, CA 90048
310-423-7933
877-223-3277

APDA Information and Referral
    Center at UCLA
Regents at the University of
    California
710 Westwood Plaza, Suite A 153
Los Angeles, CA 90095-1769
310-206-9799

San Diego
APDA Information and Referral
    Center
8555 Aero Drive
San Diego, CA 92123-1745
858-273-6763
www.sd-pc.com

Stanford
APDA Information and Referral
    Center
Stanford University Medical
    Center
Department of Neurology
300 Pasteur Drive, Room A-343
Stanford, CA 94305
866-250-2414

CONNECTICUT
New Haven
APDA Information and Referral
    Center
Hospital of Saint Raphael
Senior Services
1450 Chapel Street
New Haven, CT 06511
203-789-3936
www.ctapda.com

FLORIDA
Jacksonville
APDA Information and Referral
    Center
Mayo Clinic Jacksonville
4500 San Pablo Road
Jacksonville, FL 32224
904-953-7030

Pompano Beach
APDA Information and Referral
  Center
North Broward Medical Center
201 East Sample Road
Pompano Beach, FL 33064
800-825-2732
954-786-7316

St. Petersburg
APDA Information and Referral
  Center
Rehabilitation Institute
Edward White Hospital
1839 Central Avenue
St. Petersburg, FL 33713
727-898-2832

GEORGIA
Atlanta
APDA Information and Referral
  Center
Emory University School
  of Medicine
1841 Clifton Road NE, Room 326
Atlanta, GA 30329
404-728-6552

IDAHO
Boise
APDA Information and Referral
  Center
St. Alphonsus Regional Medical
  Center
1055 North Curtis Road
Boise, ID 83706
208-367-6569

ILLINOIS
Chicago
APDA Information and Referral
  Center
Glenbrook Hospital
2100 Pfingsten Road
Glenview, IL 60025
847-657-5787
www.Join-pdKids@lyris.parkinson
  .org.uk
www.members.aol.com/apdayp

LOUISIANA
New Orleans
APDA Information and Referral
  Center
Louisiana State University
  School of Medicine
1542 Tulane Avenue, #215
Neurology B 301116
New Orleans, LA 70112
504-568-6554

MAINE
Falmouth
APDA Information and Referral
  Center
Maine Health Learning Resource
  Center
5 Bucknam Road
Falmouth, ME 04105
207-781-1735

MARYLAND

Baltimore
APDA Information and Referral
  Center
Johns Hopkins Outpatient
  Center
Department of Neurology
601 N. Caroline Street,
  Room 5064
Baltimore, MD 21287
410-955-8795

MASSACHUSETTS

Boston
APDA Information and Referral
  Center
Boston University School of
  Medicine
Department of Neurology
720 Harrison Avenue, Suite 707
Boston, MA 02118
617-638-8466

MINNESOTA

Minneapolis
APDA Information and Referral
  Center
Abbott Northwestern Hospital
Minneapolis Neuroscience
  Institute
800 East 28th Street
Minneapolis, MN 55407
612-863-5850
888-302-7762

MISSOURI

St. Louis
APDA Information and Referral
  Center
Washington University Medical
  Center
School of Medicine
Box 8111, 660 Euclid Avenue
St. Louis, MO 63110
314-362-3299

MONTANA

Great Falls
APDA Information and Referral
  Center
Benefis Health Care—West
  Campus
500 15th Avenue South
Great Falls, MT 59405
406-455-2964
800-233-9040

NEBRASKA

Omaha
APDA Information and Referral
  Center
7701 Pacific Street, Suite 122
Omaha, NE 68114-5480
402-397-2766

NEVADA

Las Vegas
APDA Information and Referral
  Center
University of Nevada School
  of Medicine
P.O. Box 218
6029 West Charleston Road
Las Vegas, NV 89146-1116
702-464-3132

Reno
APDA Information and Referral
  Center
Veterans Administration Hospital
1000 Locust Street
Reno, NV 89520
775-328-7168

NEW JERSEY

New Brunswick
APDA Information and Referral
  Center
Robert Wood Johnson University
  Hospital
1 Robert Wood Johnson Place
New Brunswick, NJ 08901
732-745-7520

NEW MEXICO

Albuquerque
APDA Information and Referral
  Center
Healthsouth, Rehabilitation
  Hospital
7000 Jefferson NE
Albuquerque, NM 87109
800-278-5386
505-344-9478, ext. 5098

NEW YORK

Albany
The Albany Medical College
Department of Neurology A-70
215 Washington Avenue
  Extension
Albany, NY 12203
518-452-2749

Manhattan
APDA Information and Referral
  Center
New York University Medical
  Center
345 East 37th Street, Suite 317C
New York, NY 10016
212-983-1387

Old Westbury
APDA Information and Referral
  Service
NY College of Osteopathic
  Medicine
New York Institute of Technology
P.O. Box 8000, Northern
  Boulevard
Old Westbury, NY 11568
516-626-6114

Smithtown
APDA Information and Referral
  Center
St. Catherine of Siena Hospital
Route 25A
Smithtown, NY 11787
631-862-3560

Staten Island
APDA Information and Referral
  Center
Staten Island University Hospital
475 Seaview Avenue
Staten Island, NY 10305
718-226-6129

NORTH CAROLINA
Durham
APDA Information and Referral
  Center
Duke University Medical Center
Box 3333
932 Morreene Road, Suite 220
Durham, NC 27705
919-681-2033

OHIO
Cleveland
APDA Information and Referral
  Center
The Cleveland Clinic Foundation
Department of Neurology,
  Desk S10-07
9500 Euclid Avenue
Cleveland, OH 44195
216-445-8480

Cincinnati
APDA Information and Referral
  Center
University of Cincinnati Medical
  Center
231 Albert Sabin Way
Neurology, 4th Floor
ML 0525
Cincinnati, OH 45267-0525
513-558-6770
800-400-2732

OKLAHOMA
Tulsa
APDA Information and Referral
  Center
Hillcrest Medical Center System
1125 South Trenton
Tulsa, OK 74120
918-747-3747
800-364-4450

PENNSYLVANIA
Philadelphia
APDA Information and Referral
  Center
Lewis House
Crozer-Chester Medical Center
1 Medical Center Boulevard
Upland, PA 19013
610-447-2925

Pittsburgh
APDA Information and Referral
  Center
Allegheny General Hospital
420 East North Avenue, Suite 206
Pittsburgh, PA 15212
412-441-4100

RHODE ISLAND
Pawtucket
APDA Information and Referral
  Center
Memorial Hospital of Rhode
  Island
111 Brewster Street
Pawtucket, RI 02860
401-729-3165

TENNESSEE
Memphis
APDA Information and Referral
  Center
Methodist Hospital
1265 Union Avenue,
  Suite 124 Crews
Memphis, TN 38104
901-726-8141

Nashville
APDA Information and Referral
  Center
Centennial Medical Center
2300 Patterson Street
Nashville, TN 37203
615-342-4635
800-493-2842

TEXAS
Bryan
APDA Information and Referral
  Center
St. Joseph Regional Rehabilitation
  Center
1600 Joseph Drive
Bryan, TX 77802
979-821-7585

Dallas
APDA Information and Referral
  Center
Presbyterian Hospital of Dallas
Jackson Building, Ground Floor
8200 Walnut Hill Lane
Dallas, TX 75231
214-345-4224
800-725-2732
www.phscare.org

Lubbock
APDA Information and Referral
  Center
Covenant Hospital
Lubbock Diagnostic Clinic
  Building
3506 21st Street, Suite 402
Lubbock, TX 79410
806-785-2732
800-687-5498

San Antonio
APDA Information and Referral
  Center
University of Texas HSC at San
  Antonio
Division of Neurology
7703 Floyd Carl Drive, MSC 7883
San Antonio, TX 78229
210-567-4744

UTAH
Salt Lake City
APDA Information and Referral
  Center
University of Utah School of
  Medicine
Department of Neurology
50 North Medical Drive, Room
  3R 144
Salt Lake City, UT 84132
801-585-2354

VERMONT
Burlington
APDA Information and Referral
  Center
FAHC UHC Campus—
  Neurology Department
1 South Prospect Street
Burlington, VT 05401
802-847-3366
888-763-3366

VIRGINIA
Charlottesville
APDA Information and Referral
  Center
University of Virginia Health
  System
Fontaine Research Park—
  Adult Neurology
P.O. Box 801018
500 Ray C. Hunt Drive, Room 6
Charlottesville, VA 22908
434-982-1726

WASHINGTON
Seattle
APDA Information and Referral
  Center
University of Washington
Department of Neurology
Box 356465
1959 NE Pacific, RR 638
Seattle, WA 98195-6425
206-543-5369

WISCONSIN
Neenah
APDA Information and Referral
  Center
The Neurosciences Group of
  Northeast Wisconsin
200 Theda Clark Medical Plaza,
  Suite 480
Neenah, WI 54956
920-725-9373

Parkinson's Organizations in Canada

Parkinson Foundation of Canada
Nova Scotia Division Office
2786 Agricola Street, Room 214
Halifax, NS B3K 4E1
902-454-2468
800-663-2468

Parkinson Foundation of Canada
St. John's Regional Chapter
Provincial Resource Centre
P.O. Box 2568, Station C
St. John's, NF A1C 6K1
709-754-4428
800-567-7020

Parkinson Society British
  Columbia
890 West Pender Street
Vancouver, BC V6C 1K4
604-662-3240
800-668-3330
www.parkinsonsbc.com

Parkinson Society Canada
4211 Yonge Street, Suite 316
Toronto, ON M2P 2A9
416-227-9700
800-565-3000
www.parkinson.ca

Parkinson Society Canada,
  Maritime Region
5475 Spring Garden Road,
  Suite 407
Halifax, NS B3J 3T2
902-422-3656

Parkinson Society Canada,
  Ontario Division
4211 Yonge Street, Suite 316
Toronto, ON M2P 2A9
416-227-9700
800-565-3000

Parkinson Society Manitoba
825 Sherbrook Street, Suite 204
Winnipeg, MB R3A 1M5
204-786-2637

Parkinson Society Newfoundland
   & Labrador
The Ashley Building, Suite 219
31 Peet Street
St. John's, NF A1B 3W8
709-754-4428

The Parkinson's Society of Alberta
Edmonton General, Room 3Y18
11111 Jasper Avenue
Edmonton, AB T5K 0L4
780-482-8993
888-873-9801

Parkinson's Society of Ottawa
1053 Carling Avenue
Ottawa, ON K1Y 4E9
613-722-9238

Saskatchewan Parkinson's Disease
   Foundation
Box 102, 103 Hospital Drive
Saskatoon, SK S7N 0W8
306-966-8030

Societe Parkinson du Quebec
1253 McGill College, Suite 402
Montreal, QB H3B 2Y5
514-861-4422
800-720-1307 (national
   francophone line)

APPENDIX D

Sources of Adaptive Equipment, Clothing, and Other Good Things

Note: The authors have compiled this list of sources as a service to readers, but we have no personal experience with the listed businesses and organizations and make no endorsements. Many of the companies that are listed offer catalogs.

Ableware: Independent Living from Maddak, Inc., 6 Industrial Road, Pequannock, NJ 07440-1993. Telephone 973-628-7600; www.maddak .com. Bathroom, bedroom, communicating, dressing, drinking, eating, educational aids, grooming, household, kitchen, mirrors, mobility, reading and writing, recreation, exercise, and wheelchair accessories.

Access with Ease, P.O. Box 1150, Chino Valley, AZ 86323. Telephone 800-531-9479; shop.store.yahoo.com/capability/index.html. Eating, drinking, dressing, grooming, cooking, bathroom, personal care, comfort, communicating, mobility, home access, and lawn and garden.

Access to Recreation Inc., 8 Sandra Court, Newbury Park, CA 91320-4302. Telephone 800-634-4351; www.AccessTR.com. Adaptive recreational equipment, exercise equipment, and gardening tools.

Aids for Arthritis, Inc., 35 Wakefield Drive, Medford, NJ 08055. Telephone 800-654-0707; www.aidsforarthritis.com. Eating, drinking, dressing, grooming, cooking, bathroom, personal care, mobility, home access, and recreation.

Alliance for Technology Access, 2175 E. Francisco Boulevard, San Rafael, CA 94901. Telephone 415-455-4575; www.ataccess.org/default .html. Network of resource centers, developers, and vendors serving children and adults with disabilities, connecting them with technology tools.

American Self-Help Clearinghouse, Saint Clare's Health Services, 25 Pocono Road, Denville, NJ 07834-2995. Telephone 973-326-6789; 800-367-6274 NJ only; www.health.gov/nhic/NHICScripts/Entry.cfm?HRCODE =HR1681. Referrals to national and international self-help groups, as well as to local self-help clearinghouses.

Ann Morris Enterprises, Inc., 890 Fams Court, East Meadow, NY 11554-5101. Telephone 516-292-9232 and 800-454-3175; www.annmorris .com. Eating, drinking, dressing, grooming, cooking, bathroom, personal care, communicating, mobility, home access, and exercise.

Attainment Company, P.O. Box 930160, Verona, WI 53593-0160. Telephone 800-327-4269; www.attainmentcompany.com. Eating, drinking, cooking, communicating, and home access.

The Best 25 Catalog Resources for Making Life Easier by Shelley Peterman Schwarz. $3, c/o DMA, 1111 19th Street NW, Suite 1100, Washington, DC 20036. Telephone 202-955-5030; www.makinglifeeasier.com/books/b25.html.

Bruce Medical Supply, P.O. Box 9166, Waltham, MA 02454-9166. Telephone 800-225-8446; www.brucemedical.com. Eating, drinking, dressing, grooming, personal care, communicating, and managing home health care.

Comfort Home, 189 Frelinghuysen Avenue, Newark, NJ 07114-1595. Telephone 800-359-7701; www.comforthouse.com. Dressing, grooming, cooking, bathroom, personal care, mobility, home access, exercise, lawn, and garden.

Dynamic Living Inc., 428 Hayden Station Road, Windsor, CT 06095-1302. Telephone 888-940-0605; www.dynamic-living.com. Cooking, general aids, clothing, automotive, as well as hearing and speaking aids.

Easy Street, P.O. Box 146, Foxboro, MA 02035. Telephone 800-959-EASY; www.easystreetco.com. Eating, drinking, dressing, grooming, cooking, bathroom, personal care, communicating, mobility, home access, and exercise.

ENDependence Center of Northern Virginia, Inc., 3100 Clarendon Boulevard, Arlington, VA 22201. Telephone 703-525-3268; www.ecnv .org. Information on adaptive clothing and accessories.

Enrichments, Sammons-Preston, Inc. (a subsidiary of Bissell Health Care), P.O. Box 5071, Bollingbrook, IL 60440. Telephone 800-323-5547; www.sammonspreston.com. Eating, drinking, dressing, grooming, cooking, personal care, communicating, mobility, home access, exercise, wheelchairs, and wheelchair accessories.

Fashion Ease, 1541 60th Street, Brooklyn, NY 11219-9958. Telephone 800-221-8929; www.fashionease.com. By M&M Healthcare Apparel Co. Clothing with elastic, snaps, buttons, zippers, or Velcro closures.

Hard-to-Find-Tools, Brookstone, 1655 Bassford Drive, Mexico, MO 65265. Telephone 800-926-7000; www.brookstone.com. Dressing, grooming, cooking, bathroom, personal care, home access, lawn, and gardening.

Independent Living Aids, 27 East Mall, Plainview, NY 11803-4404. Telephone 800-537-2188; www.independentliving.com. Eating, drinking, dressing, grooming, cooking, bathroom, personal care, communicating, mobility, home access, and many items for people with low vision.

International Cushioned Products, 9505 Haldame Road, Kelowna, BC V4V 2KS. Telephone 800-TUB-SOFT; www.softbathtubs.com. Soft bathtubs.

Lighthouse, Inc., 111 E. 59th Street, New York, NY 10022-1202. Telephone 800-829-0500; www.lighthouse.org. Personal care, communicating, leisure, recreation.

Maxi-Aids, Inc., 42 Executive Boulevard, Farmingdale, NY 11735. Telephone 800-522-6294 or 631-752-0521; www.maxiaids.com. Eating, drinking, cooking, bathroom, personal care, communicating, mobility, and home access.

MedicAlert Foundation International, 2323 Colorado Avenue, Turlock, CA 95382. Telephone 888-633-4298; (outside the United States 209-668-3333); www.medicalert.org. First year is $35, $20 each year thereafter; provides a bracelet or a necklace that alerts emergency medical personnel to your medical condition and gives them access to medical information and the names of physicians and relatives.

National Association of Area Agencies on Aging, 927 15th Street NW, Washington, DC 20005. Telephone 202-296-8130; www.n4a.org. Umbrella organization for 655 area agencies on aging, which coordinates services to help older individuals be able to remain in their homes. The Web site has links to local agencies on aging.

S & S Worldwide, 75 Mill Street, Colchester, CT 06415-0513. Telephone 800-243-9232; www.snswwide.com. Eating, drinking, dressing, grooming, cooking, bathroom, personal care, home access, and exercise.

Sears Home Health Care, 3737 Grader Street, Suite 110, Garland, TX 75041. Telephone 800-326-1750. Dressing, grooming, bathroom, personal care, mobility, home access, and exercise.

Self Care Catalog, 104 Challenger Drive, Portland, TN 37148-1716. Telephone 800-345-3371; www.selfcare.com. Cooking, dressing, grooming, bathroom, personal care, mobility, and exercise.

Speech Booster, P.O. Box 1810, Diamond Spring, CA 95619. Telephone 800-224-5141. Portable, battery-powered amplifier; can be worn in public settings to help others hear the wearer.

Sunshine Comfort Wear, 4555 Renaissance Parkway, Cleveland, OH 44128. Telephone 888-595-9888. Clothing for men and women with elastic, snaps, cutout seats, or side zippers.

Wardrobe Wagon, Telephone 800-WW-CARES. Clothing with snap or zipper closures.

Bibliography for Chapter 8: Medications and Therapies

Abrams, R. "ECT for Parkinson's Disease" (Editorial). *American Journal of Psychiatry* 146, no. 11 (1989): 1391–93.

Altman, L. K. "Nerve Protein Raises Hope for Paralyzed." *New York Times*, January 18, 1990, B7.

Birkmayer, W., et al. "Deprenyl Leads to Prolongation of L-Dopa Efficacy in Parkinson's Disease." *Mod. Probl. Pharmacopsychiat.* 19 (1983): 170–76.

Bishop, Jerry E. "Scientists Grow Human Brain Cells in Laboratory Dishes for the First Time." *Wall Street Journal*, May 4, 1990, B4.

Borek, C. "Parkinson's Defense." *Nutrition Science News.* The Nutritional Journal of Natural Products Research and Innovation, May 2001; www.newhope.com/nutritionsciencenews/NSN_backs/May_01/parkinsons.cfm.

Calne, D. "Letter of Concern." *Parkinson Network* (Newsletter of the Parkinson Foundation of Canada) (April 1990): 2–3.

Chance, J. "Clinical Follow-Up of Post-Pallidotomy and Neurotransplantation Patients." Presentation at a symposium sponsored by the Neurosciences Institute and Good Samaritan Hospital, Los Angeles, November 2–3, 1996.

Donn, J. "Parkinson's Patient Heartened by Stem Cell Compromise." Associated Press, August 10, 2001.

Douyon, R., et al. "ECT and Parkinson's Disease Revisited: A 'Naturalist' Study." *American Journal of Psychiatry* 146, no. 11 (1989): 1451–55.

Durso, Raymon. "Pharmacology of Parkinson Disease." (Unpublished paper.)

Duvoisin, R. C. "Etiology of Parkinson's Disease: Current Concepts." *Clin. Neuropharmacol.* 9, suppl. 1 (1986): S3–S11.

———. *Parkinson's Disease: A Guide for Patient and Family*. New York: Raven Press, 1978.

Duvoisin, R. C., et al. "Discussion." *Clin. Neuropharmacol.* 9, suppl. 1 (1986): S13–S21.

Feldman, R. G., and M. C. Lannon. "Parkinson Disease: Individualizing Therapy." *Hospital Practice* 20 (1985): 80A–80FF.

Foreman, J. "Surgery and Transplants Show New Promise." *Boston Globe*, June 19, 1995.

Freed, C. R., et al. "Transplantation of Human Fetal Dopamine Cells for Parkinson's Disease: Results at 1 Year." *Archives of Neurology* 47 (1990): 505–11.

Friedrich, M. J. "Fetal Pig Neural Cells for Parkinson Disease." *Journal of the American Medical Association* 282, no. 23 (December 15, 1999): 2198–2199.

Gale, K. "Brain Stimulation Benefit for Parkinson's Lasts." Reuter's Health, November 13, 2003.

Goetz, C. G. "Brain Transplants in Parkinson's Disease: Where Do We Stand?" *United Parkinson Foundation Newsletter* 2, part 2 (1989): 1–2.

Goetz, C. G., et al. "Multicenter Study of Autologous Adrenal Medullary Transplantation to the Corpus Striatum in Patients with Advanced Parkinson's Disease." *New England Medicine* 320 (1989): 337–41.

Golbe, L. I., et al. "Deprenyl in the Treatment of Symptom Fluctuations in Advanced Parkinson's Disease." *Clin. Neuropharmacol.* 11, no. 1 (1988): 45–55.

Guyer, R. L. "Neural Graft for Parkinson's Disease." *This Week in Science* (February 2, 1990): 511.

Henke, J. "Parkinson's Disease: New Treatments Slow Onslaught of Symptoms." *FDA Consumer Magazine*. Food and Drug Administration, July–August 1998; www.fda.gov/fdac/features/1998/498_pd.html.

Knoll, J. "Role of B-Type Monoamine Oxidase Inhibition in the Treatment of Parkinson's Disease: An Update." In *Movement Disorders*, ed. by N. S. Shah and A. G. Donald. New York: Plenum, 1986, 53–81.

Kolata, G. "Fetal Tissue Seems to Aid Parkinson Patient." *New York Times*, February 2, 1990, A1, A20.

————. "New Drug Slows Parkinson's, Study Confirms." *New York Times*, November 16, 1980, B18.

Lees, A., ed. *Deprenyl in Parkinson's Disease: Guidelines for Clinicians.* (Proceedings of panel discussion in San Francisco on October 18, 1987.) London: Royal Society of Medicine Services Ltd., 1988.

Lewin, R. "Big First Scored with Nerve Diseases." *Science* 245 (1989): 467–68.

————. "Clinical Trial for Parkinson's Disease?" *Science* 230 (1985): 527–28.

LeWitt, P. A. "New Perspectives in the Treatment of Parkinson's Disease." *Clin. Neuropharmacol.* 9, suppl. 1 (1986): S37–S46.

LeWitt, P. A., et al. "Discussion." *Clin. Neuropharmacol.* 9, suppl. 1 (1986): S47–S54.

Lieberman, A. N. "Adrenal Grafts Transplanted into the Brain as a Treatment for Parkinson's." *APDA Newsletter* (Fall 1987): 1, 5–6.

————. "Brain Transplants: A Report on Experimental Treatments for Parkinson's Disease." *APDA Newsletter* (Winter/Spring 1988): 1–2.

————. "Curing Parkinson's Disease in Our Lifetime: Part 3." *Parkinson Report* (quarterly of the National Parkinson Foundation, Inc.) (Fall 2000): 10–12.

————. "The Ninth International Symposium on Parkinson's Disease." *APDA Newsletter* (Winter 1988/1989): 1, 4, 6.

————. "Treatment of Parkinson's Disease." *APDA Newsletter* (Spring 1989): 2.

Lieberman, A. N., et al. *Parkinson's Disease Handbook.* New York: American Parkinson Disease Association. (Undated.)

Lindvall, O., et al. "Grafts of Fetal Dopamine Neurons Survive and Improve Motor Function in Parkinson's Disease." *Science* 247 (1990): 574–77.

Lukazewski, A. "Pharmacologic Management Approach to Parkinsonism." *AgeNet*, October 27, 2003; www.agenet.agenet.com.

Luo, J., et al. "Subthalamic GAD Gene Therapy in a Parkinson's Disease Rat Model." *Science* 298, no. 5592 (October 11, 2002): 425–29.

Marx, J. "Fetal Nerve Grafts Show Promise in Parkinson's." *Research News* (February 2, 1990): 529.

Michelmore, P. "Six Who Dared: The Parkinson's Pioneers." *Reader's Digest* (June 1988): 75–84.

Muenter, M. D. "Pharmacotherapy: Problems and Practices." *Clin. Neuropharmacol.* 9, suppl. 1 (1986): S23–S27.

Muenter, M. D., et al. "Discussion." *Clin. Neuropharmacol.* 9, suppl. 1 (1986): S29–S36.

O'Neill, R., and P. Kidd. "Fetal Tissue Transplants Go to Clinical Trial." *Parkinson Network* (Newsletter of the Parkinson Foundation of Canada) (April 1990): 1, 3.

Pearson, H. "Stem Cell Hopes Double." *Nature* (June 21, 2002); www.nature.com/nsu/020617/020617-11.html.

Polsby, M. "You, Your Doctor, and Parkinson's Disease." Transcription of a talk at Camp Maria, 1986.

Rasmussen, K. G., et al. "Electroconvulsive Therapy and Newer Modalities for the Treatment of Medication-Refractory Mental Illness." *Mayo Clinic Proceedings* #77 (Mayo Foundation for Medical Education and Research) (2002): 552–56.

Recer, P. "Bush Backs Limited Embryonic Stem Cell Research." *Associated Press*, August 10, 2001.

———. "Gene Therapy to Be Tried for Late-State Parkinson's Disease Patients." *Associated Press*, October 11, 2002.

Rezak, M. "Comtan (Entacapone): A New Catechol-O-Methyltransferase Inhibitor Is Released." *Young Parkinson's Newsletter* of the American Parkinson's Disease Association, Inc. (Spring 2000): 1.

St. Hilaire, M. "Dopamine Agonists in the Early Treatment of Parkinson's Disease." *Parkinson's Today & Tomorrow* (quarterly of the Massachusetts Chapter of the APDA) (Winter 2002): 2–3.

———. "Parkinson's Disease: New Possibilities." *Health Confidential* (October 1989): 3.

———. "The Use of Deprenyl in Parkinson's Disease." *Progress Notes: A Report from the Parkinson's Disease Center at Boston University Medical Center* (July 1989): 1.

Shoulson, I., et al. (Parkinson Study Group.) "Effect of Deprenyl on the Progression of Disability in Early Parkinson's Disease." *New England Journal of Medicine* 321, no. 20 (1989): 1364–71.

Shults, C. W., et al. "Evidence of Coenzyme Q10 in Early Parkinson Disease." *Archives of Neurology* 59 (2002):1541–50.

Snyder, B. "New Surgery Liberates Parkinson's Patients." *Nashville Tennessean*, May 21, 2000.

Steinberg, D. "Gene Therapists Aim for Parkinson's Disease." *The Scientist* 15, no. 19 (October 1, 2001): 18.

Tetrud, J. W., and J. W. Langston. "The Effect of Deprenyl (Selegiline) on the Natural History of Parkinson's Disease." *Science* 245 (1989): 519–22.

Teychenne, P. F. "Low-Dose Parlodel (Bromocriptine Mesylate) Therapy in Parkinson's Disease." Report prepared by Sandoz, Inc., 1981.

Weiner, W. J. "Non-Motor Symptoms in Parkinson's Disease." *NPF Parkinson Report* 10, no. 1, (1989): 1–4.

Weiss, R. "Bypassing the Ban." *Science News* 136 (1989): 378–79.

———. "Coalition against Therapeutic Substitution." *Parkinson's Disease Foundation Newsletter* (Autumn 1988): 1.

———. "DATATOP Study Confirms Deprenyl's Efficacy in Fighting the Progression of Parkinson's Disease." Release by National Institute of Neurological Disorders and Stroke, National Institutes of Health (January 20, 1993).

———. *Early Addition of Parlodel*. (Pamphlet). East Hanover, N. J.: Sandoz Pharmaceuticals Corp.

———. *Eldepryl Investigators Product Profile*. Denville, N. J.: Somerset Pharmaceuticals, Inc.

———. "Embryonic Mouse Stem Cells Reduce Symptoms in Model for Parkinson's Disease." Release by National Institute of Neurological Disorders and Stroke, National Institutes of Health, June 20, 2002.

———. "Fetal Cell Recipient Showing Improvements." *Science News* 137 (1990): 70.

———. "Fetal Tissue Research—HHS Ruling." *Parkinson's Disease Foundation Newsletter* (Summer 1988): 1.

———. "Foundation Awards $4.4 Million in Grants for PD Cell Line Initiative." Release by Michael J. Fox Foundation for Parkinson's Research, March 2002; www.michaeljfox.org/news/press.

———. "Gene Therapy for Parkinson's." *BBC NEWS, World Edition*, October 10, 2002; www.news.bbc.co.uk/2/hi/health/2316613.stm.

———. "Genetic Study of Parkinson's Disease." *APDA Newsletter* (Winter/Spring 1988): 5.

———. "High Dosage Vitamins E and C in Early Parkinson's Disease." *APDA Newsletter* (Spring 1989): 5. (Based on Fahn, S., New York Academy of Sciences, "Vitamin E. Biochemistry and Health Implications," October 31–November 2, 1988.)

———. "Hope of Parkinson's 'Cure'." *BBC NEWS, World Edition*, October 27, 2000; www.news.bbc.co.uk/2/hi/health/991965.stm.

———. "The Michael J. Fox Foundation Announces Research Fellowships." Release by Michael J. Fox Foundation for Parkinson's Research, August 2002; www.michaeljfox.org/news/press.

———. "The Michael J. Fox Foundation for Parkinson's Research to Fund Search for Parkinson's Biomarker." Release by Michael J. Fox Foundation for Parkinson's Research, April 8, 2002; www.michaeljfox .org/news/press.

———. "Now Available, New Stalevo Addresses Top Parkinson's Disease Concern." *The National Parkinson Foundation, Inc.*, September 16, 2003.

———. "Parkinson's Disease: Innovative Approaches Offer New Hope." *Lahey Clinic Health Magazine* (Winter 2000): 1–3.

———. *Parkinson's Disease: Progress, Promise, and Hope!* New York: Parkinson's Disease Foundation, 1984.

———. "Parkinson's Patients Look to Gene Therapy." Associated Press, *CNN.com/HEALTH*. Cable News Network LP, LLP, October 11, 2002.

———. "Pharmacologic Advancements in the Treatment of Parkinson's Disease." *Parkinson's Nursing News* 1, no. 1 (Spring 1999): 1–4, 6–7.

———. "Report: Vitamin E, Parkinson's Drug Slow Alzheimer's Disease." *CNN Interactive*. Cable News Network, Inc. April, 23, 1997.

———. "Shock Therapy's Parkinsonian Potential." *Science News* 136 (1989): 381.

———. "Shrink-Wrapped Transplants for Parkinson's." *Science* 248 (1990): 816.

———. "United Parkinson Foundation Brain Implant Workshop." *Parkinson's Disease Foundation Newsletter* (Summer 1988): 3.

———. "Update on Surgery for Parkinson's, Taken from Dr. Fahn's Open House Talk." *Parkinson's Disease Foundation Newsletter* (Summer 1988): 1–2.

———. "Vitamin E and Parkinson's Disease." *APDA Newsletter* (Spring 1989): 3. (Based on Factor, S. A., et al., New York Academy of Sciences, "Vitamin E: Biochemistry and Health Implications," October 31–November 2, 1988.)

———. "Year-End Summary Related to Parkinson's Disease." *National Parkinson Foundation Newsletter* (February 1989): 1–4.

General Bibliography

(Not including sources for chapter 8)

Beaver, L. L., and C. H. Markham. *How to Start a Parkinson's Disease Community Support Group*. New York: American Parkinson Disease Association. (Undated.)

Bloise, J. "Parkinson's Doesn't Stop Him." *Eagle-Tribune*, December 13, 1998.

Burtis, G., et al. *Applied Nutrition and Diet Therapy*. Philadelphia: Saunders, 1988, 76–77, 82, 784–87.

Carter, J. H. "Nutrition: An Important Compliment [sic] to PD Management," *Parkinson's Nursing News* 1, no. 2 (Summer 1999).

Cote, L., and G. Riedel. *Exercises for the Parkinson Patient, with Hints for Daily Living*. New York: Parkinson's Disease Foundation. (Undated.)

Coyne, J. *Social Support, an Interactional View*. New York: John Wiley & Sons, 1990.

Cunningham, L. O. "How to Talk to Your Doctor." *Woman's Day* (August 4, 1987).

Drake, C. J. *How to Start a Parkinson's Support Group*. Newport Beach, Calif.: Parkinson's Educational Program. (Undated.)

Duvoisin, R. C. *Parkinson's Disease: A Guide for Patient and Family*, 2nd ed. New York: Raven Press, 1984.

Elliott, K. "Nutrition and Parkinsonism." Unpublished paper presented at a workshop. (Undated.)

Flapan, M. "Living with Parkinson's: What Can You Do for Yourself . . . ?" *Parkinson's Disease Foundation Newsletter* (Autumn 1989): 2–3.

Fox, M. J. *Lucky Man: A Memoir*. New York: Hyperion, 2002.

Goleman, D. "Advising People in Distress: What to Say and What Not to Say." *New York Times*, February 15, 1990, B19.

Hauser, R., and T. Zesiewicz. *Parkinson's Disease: Questions and Answers*, 2nd ed. Coral Springs, Fla.: Merit Publishing International, 1999.

Kondracke, M. *Saving Milly: Love, Politics, and Parkinson's Disease*. New York: Public Affairs, 2001.

Levin, E. "Mirror, Mirror on the Wall" (Flyer). Newport Beach, Calif.: Parkinson's Educational Program. (Undated.)

Levin, S. B., and E. B. Montgomery. *Coping with Parkinson's Disease.* (Pamphlet.) St. Louis: Jewish Hospital and Greater St. Louis Chapter, American Parkinson Disease Association, 1986.

Lieberman, A. N., et al. *Parkinson Disease Handbook: A Guide for Patients and Their Families*. American Parkinson Disease Association. (Undated.)

Loftus, S. "Get Up and Go! An Exercise Program for People with Parkinson's Disease." *American Journal of Nursing* (February 1988): 254.

Maroney, E., "Doctor Offers Straight Talk on Living with Parkinson's." *The Barnstable Patriot*, August 3, 2000.

Paulson, G. W., and J. L. Howard. (Untitled essay on sexuality in Parkinson's disease.) *UPF Newsletter* 4, part 2 (1985): 1–7.

Perry, L. "Principles of Application of the Low-Protein Diet." *Progress Notes*, Parkinson Disease Center at Boston University Medical Center (February 1990): 2–3.

Pincus, J. H., and K. Barry. "Protein Redistribution Diet for Parkinson's Disease." (Diet of the Yale University Hospital Parkinson's Clinic.)

Polsby, M. "You, Your Doctor, and Parkinson's Disease." Transcription of a talk given in 1986.

Riley, D., and A. E. Lang. "Practical Application of a Low-Protein Diet for Parkinson's Disease." *Neurology 38* (1988): 1026–31.

Robinson, M. B. *Equipment and Suggestions to Help the Patient with Parkinson's Disease in the Activities of Daily Living*. New York: American Parkinson Disease Association, 1989.

St. Hilaire, M. "The Use of Low-Protein Diet in Parkinson's Disease." *Progress Notes*, Parkinson's Disease Center at Boston University Medical Center (February 1990): 1–2.

Strong, Maggie. *Mainstay: For the Well Spouse of the Chronically Ill*. New York: Little, Brown & Company, 1989.

Vosskuehler, C. *Home Exercise Program for Patients with Parkinson's Disease*. New York: American Parkinson Disease Association. (Undated.)

———. "Neuropsychology Clinic Opens at Welkind Rehabilitation Hospital." *Neighbor News* (Denville, N.J.), January 3, 1990.

———. *Speech Problems and Swallowing Problems in Parkinson's Disease*. New York: American Parkinson Disease Association, 1989.

———. "Woman Refuses to Let Parkinson's Keep Her Down for Long." *Huber Heights Courier*, March 2, 1988, 5.

Index